Foundations of
Curative Eurythmy

You may also be interested in

Anthroposophical Care for the Elderly
Annegret Camps, Brigitte Hagenhoff and Ada van der Star

Anthroposophical Therapeutic Speech
Barbara Denjean-von Stryk and Dietrich von Bonin

Biographical Work: The Anthroposophical Basis
Gudrun Burkhard

*Compresses and other Therapeutic Applications:
A Handbook from the Ita Wegman Clinic*
Monika Fingado

Foundations of Curative Eurythmy
Margarete Kirchner-Bockholt

The Physiology of Eurythmy Therapy
Hans-Broder von Laue and Elke E von Laue

Rhythmic Einreibung: A Handbook from the Ita Wegman Clinic
Monika Fingado

The Background to Anthroposophical Therapeutic Speech
Edited by Dietrich von Bonin

FOUNDATIONS OF CURATIVE EURYTHMY

Margarete Kirchner-Bockholt

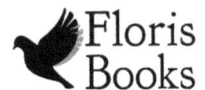

Translated by Janet Wood

First published in English in 1977 by Rudolf Steiner Press
This edition published in 2004 by Floris Books
Fourth printing 2018

Originally published in German under the title *Grundelemente der Heil-Eurythmie* by Philosophisch-Anthroposophischer Verlag am Goetheanum, Dornach, Switzerland in 1962
© Philosophisch-Anthroposophischer Verlag am Goetheanum
This translation © 1992 Floris Books

All rights reserved. No part of this publication may be reproduced without the prior permission of Floris Books, Edinburgh
www.florisbooks.co.uk

British Library CIP Data available
ISBN 978-086315-466-9
Printed by Lightning Source

Contents

Preface   vii

Introduction   1

Part 1

1. Curative Eurythmy   5
2. The Alphabet   11
3. Practical Application   16
4. The Vowels   21
5. Vowel Sequences   53
6. Basic Exercises   61
7. The Cosmic Aspect of the Vowels   72

Part 2

8. Vowels and Consonants   81
9. The Consonants   88
10. Consonantal and Zodiacal Forces in the Human Form   133
11. Consonant Sequences   151

12	Consonants and Vowels in Mixed Sequences	164
	Epilogue	172
	Appendix	173
	Bibliography	174
	Index	175

Preface

We are indebted to Rudolf Steiner for curative eurythmy as an important factor in therapy.

Eurythmy as an art, and also in the educational field, had already been developed to a considerable extent by the year 1921, when from the medical profession, and also from some eurythmists, questions were put to Rudolf Steiner as to whether or not certain eurythmic movements could have a direct healing effect. The eurythmists Erna Wolfram and Elizabeth Baumann were especially tireless in their efforts in this field.

In reply to these questions Rudolf Steiner gave a course of lectures in April 1921 for doctors and medical students, in which he developed the basic principles of curative eurythmy. He modified the movements of eurythmy, and the practical exercises thus created were demonstrated for the first time by the two people mentioned above. In this way he laid the foundation for a therapy of eurythmic movements which is especially important for anthroposophical medicine. During the next few years he was able to add considerably to the exercises with indications given in actual cases of illness.

In the year 1922 Rudolf Steiner entrusted Frl. Dr (med.) Grete Bockholt with the development of curative eurythmy and the training of curative eurythmists. As a doctor, she had herself taken a course in eurythmy and since then worked indefatigably at its theoretical and practical development. The present book contains a synopsis of what has been given in the curriculum of innumerable training courses.

On the one hand it is intended as a guide for curative eurythmists in their work, and on the other hand—and this appears to be particularly important—it should give the general medical practitioner an opportunity of becoming thoroughly acquainted with this branch of therapy.

May this book help curative eurythmy to play a part of ever-increasing importance in anthroposophical medicine. At the same time this would be the most realistic way of showing our gratitude to Rudolf Steiner.

M.P. van Deventer
1962

Introduction

In April 1921 a course of lectures for doctors was given at the Goetheanum in Dornach. Within this framework Rudolf Steiner gave the first six lectures on curative eurythmy to doctors and invited eurythmists. In these lectures all the basic curative eurythmy exercises were shown. A seventh lecture was added for doctors only, dealing more with the physiological side of curative eurythmy. In the following year, at a medical conference in Stuttgart, once again at the urgent request of the doctors, Rudolf Steiner gave additional material on the subject of curative eurythmy.

A start was made by putting the instructions into practice in the Waldorf school in Stuttgart and in the then existing clinics and nursing homes in Stuttgart and Arlesheim. Astonishing discoveries were made of the many possibilities opened up by these new methods of healing. Then in the years 1923–4 the curative educational work was begun and curative eurythmy assumed very special significance as a healing factor in the treatment of children in need of special care. During the 40 years which have elapsed since its inception, a great deal of experience has been gained in the schools, curative institutions, nursing homes and also in the private practices of many doctors. Thus curative eurythmy has become a new therapy. In the years when it was still possible to put questions to Rudolf Steiner he gave much practical advice in actual cases. Then, however, we were faced with the problem of reaching the point, through observation and study, of being ourselves able to apply the right sound in precisely the right way in a specific case.

Since that time several hundred curative eurythmists have been trained and many of them are actively trying to satisfy an ever-growing demand.

From all those who did not take part in the very beginnings of curative eurythmy, the urgent request has been repeatedly expressed for the publication of the basic principles and for an authentic collection of the subject matter given by Rudolf Steiner. For naturally, in the ordinary course of curative eurythmy practice new exercises are always being devised as they arise out of the pattern of a particular illness. These are not as suitable for study material as those actually given by Rudolf Steiner. Therefore an attempt has been made to compile a collection of the exercises he gave. A sound basis is provided for the further development of curative eurythmy if one can return again and again to Rudolf Steiner's original suggestions. The Curative Eurythmy Course contains all the rudiments which we need for the application and further expansion of this new therapy. Curative eurythmy is only at the beginning of its development and therefore everything that is described in this book can only be regarded as a stimulus to further study.

Two important therapeutic fields of application for curative eurythmy have intentionally not been dealt with. For many years exercises which are specially for eye complaints have been used with great success. This branch of curative eurythmy has been built up particularly by Dr Ilse Knauer and there is hope that she will herself write something about it.

The vast field of curative tone eurythmy also offers great possibilities for therapy. Rudolf Steiner gave only a few indications. The more the inner mobility of the human being declines, the more necessary will the relaxing, healing forces of tone eurythmy be needed to create harmony. Together with Frl. van der Pals I have been able to work out the first rudiments which have been passed on in training courses. It would be premature to make this public. Some eurythmists, e.g. Frl. Else Sittel and Frl. Trude Thetter, continue to work further in the field of curative tone eurythmy.

I am very grateful to Frl. Lily Herz for her help in the preparation of this book. Her offer of help gave the first impulse for the book which was urgently requested at a recapitulation course of curative eurythmy in July 1960.

I would also like to express my thanks to the curative eurythmists at the clinic in Arlesheim, Frl. Dr Sattler and Frau Erica Muller, for their ever-willing help; also to Frau Christel Suchantke for her drawings and illustrations.

Dr (med.) M. Kirchner-Bockholt
1962

Editor's note: Quotations not otherwise marked are from the Curative Eurythmy Course (see *Curative Eurythmy*, eight lectures, Dornach, 12-18 April 1921, Stuttgart 28th October 1922), or
Eurythmy as Visible Speech, the fundamental course on speech eurythmy (15 lectures, Dornach, 24 June–12 July 1924). Some lecture dates have been added to the text in brackets.

PART 1

CHAPTER 1

Curative Eurythmy

Curative eurythmy may be regarded as a metamorphosis of artistic eurythmy. This new art of movement was inaugurated by Rudolf Steiner and had its first beginnings in 1912.

Eurythmy is visible speech and is thereby differentiated from dance or mime. The elements of speech, vowels and consonants, which originate in the larynx and the organs connected with it, are transformed into movements and thus become visible. In the same way as our speech organism makes certain definite gestures when we say 'Ah' or 'OO', or when a consonant is formed by the lips or palate, so do the gestures of eurythmy follow certain fixed laws which belong to that particular sound and can express that one sound only. The configurations of the movement are not arbitrary; they give full scope to the artistic creation of movement just as in the case of our speech.

The human being can only bring forth the sounds of speech with which he is endowed, because the divine creative Word has formed the human organism through many evolutions of the earth in such a way that the microcosmic Word can sound forth in answer to the macrocosmic Word. So in eurythmy too, the creative Word speaks through the human form and all the movements within its capacity. The art of eurythmy, as it was given by Rudolf Steiner, is a creation of the spirit which leads one to the human being because its instrument is the human organism itself. In man are to be found revealed the same forces and forms of movement which are also found everywhere in the universe and in nature, but which are only hidden from our physical senses because they belong to the etheric worlds in which the only creative activity of the Word is revealed.

If we study all the possibilities of human movements as a whole, we can divide it, to begin with, into voluntary and involuntary movements.

The voluntary movements are carried out by the skeletal muscles consisting of striated muscle fibres. The involuntary movements are carried out by the plain muscles. The movements of our inner organs, the intestines and the blood vessels, belong to the involuntary movements. Thus our movements are not of a uniform character.

By means of our limbs we move about on the earth, carry out our actions and express our feelings in gestures of sympathy and antipathy. Everything we do that is an outward expression of our inner willing and feeling has to make use of these limb movements.

Whether we walk or stand, sit or lie, we are immersed in the influences of the earth, such as the force of gravity. All mechanical laws are expressions of this physical world to which we are subject in every movement of our limbs. 'The human being unites himself with certain earthly forces by orientating his organism to these forces. He learns to stand upright and walk, to find his balance in these earthly forces by means of his arms and hands. These forces do *not* work in from the cosmos, but are *purely* earthly forces.'

The involuntary movements are different; they are of a cosmic nature. They are withdrawn from our conscious experience and therefore from our free will. Because of this we are in another realm of movement, namely, the etheric.

In the book, *Fundamentals of Therapy* by Rudolf Steiner and Ita Wegman, those forces of gravity which work outwards from the earth are called 'out-raying' forces, and those which work inwards from the outermost reaches of the universe are called the 'in-raying' forces.

We have to imagine the whole world of movement active in the forces coming from the periphery, and which live not in heaviness but in buoyancy, as being far more diverse than all our physically visible movements put together. We do not see these cosmic movements but we know them by their effects on the fluid secretions, the circulation, and on all the movements of the inner organs. Rudolf Steiner makes this wealth of invisible movements, which come from the surrounding universe, visible to us in the eurythmic gestures of the sounds, especially those of the consonants.

The forms of movements which, as a basis, lie within all organically living nature are revealed to us when we occupy ourselves with each sound and practise it and get to know it. The enveloping gesture of 'B', the swelling, growth-furthering power of 'L', the rolling, vibrating 'R', are the creative language of the ebbing and flowing etheric world which lies behind the frozen world of the senses.

The impulse of the vowel to movement, in which man expresses his own being, springs from the world that is the home of our astral body. How do these movements stand in relation to the two realms of the physical and etheric worlds which we have been describing?

The astral realms, whence the vowels sound forth to us, find their visible expression in the stars which sparkle in the night sky and are like windows through which forces come to us from worlds beyond space and time. They are inward-turning forces. In embryology they are known to us in the gastrula formation: they are forces of the astral world flowing into our physical and etheric world, and create something inward as opposed to what is external. The realm of the inner organs which is not yet found in the plant kingdom, but appears first in animals and man, is an imprint of the starry world—an 'inner world system', as described by Rudolf Steiner in his lecture-course *Occult Physiology*. Our soul lives in the rhythm of this inner and outer star world—a rhythm which can only exist when there is a connection between an outer and an inner world. We shall see later in more detail how the vowels are connected with the organs of our inner world-system (see Chapter 7).

Thus we have a third sphere: forces streaming from the astral worlds which create movement and rhythm in us.

It can be said of these three kinds of forces: 'the "out-raying" forces are the earthly ones, the "in-raying" ones are the earth-encompassing forces, while in the astral forces we have something which is above both the other two. These forces make the earth itself into a heavenly body, a star. The earth separates itself off from the universe through the physical forces; through the etheric forces it lays itself open to the influences of the universe; through the astral forces it becomes an independent individuality in the universe.' [*Fundamentals of Therapy*.] What has been said here about the earth is true also for animal and man.

We have described three different kinds of movement, in the physical, the etheric and the astral. The fourth impulse to movement comes from the power of our ego. The ego-power works as movement only in man. The upright movement—the ability to stand erect between heaven and earth—is the attribute of the ego in man. Because of this upright movement of the ego all other movements are altered.

The upright gait of the human being comes from the fact that he is continually recreating a balance. With every step the ego-organization comes to terms with the force of gravity and holds itself in balance. The ego creates a balance between buoyancy and heaviness in the realm of the fluid man. In the realm of the air-man the manifestations of soul in the expressions and impulses of the astral body are brought into rhythmic balance at the point where the circulation and breathing rhythm meet.

For the practice of curative eurythmy, a continuing study of the anthroposophical aspects of the human being is necessary. For only through this can we learn how the various parts of the human being are active in human movements.

The metabolic-limb system is the real movement system. The movements of the limbs and the digestive organs adjust themselves to the rhythm of the blood circulation. This, in its turn, is regulated by the breathing processes which mediate between the rhythms of the inner and outer worlds. Thus in the chest region we have a middle system of rhythmical movement processes. Upwards, towards the head, which is the centre of the nerve-sense activity, all movement ceases, comes to rest. This threefoldness in the human being gives us an insight into how movements come about at all. We shall not discuss here the perpetual thesis that certain groups of nerve fibres are regarded as motor nerves, that is to say, they are viewed as the cause of the movements. We shall rather try to show how the motive power is brought about by a working together of the threefold human being in head, chest and limbs.

These three systems are formed in ways very different from each other. The spherical form of the head is the most bony—the flat bones of the skull envelop the brain. We must reckon the whole circumference of the outer physical world as part of the head which is the centre of the nerves and sense-organs, since it is here, in the nerve-sense system, that this outer, physical world is perceived.

In the middle system we see from the skeleton how the rhythmic element works in the arrangement of the ribs and the intercostal muscles.

In the limbs the bones are inside, surrounded by muscles and blood vessels. The functioning of the will is served by the muscles through the flexors and extensors which make possible the great diversity of movements. Here the bones are merely supports. Rudolf Steiner compares them to radii which unite in man from all sides: 'The limb system has its centre in the whole circumference. The centre of the limb system is indeed a sphere; namely, the opposite of a point, the surface of a sphere. The centre is really everywhere; hence, you can turn in every direction and radii ray in from all sides. They unite themselves with you.' [*Study of Man*.] This is a very unusual point of view. But it enables us to understand the connection between our own movements and those of the cosmos, and this is of special importance for eurythmy. Just as there is around our head a universe which we can observe calmly with our head, we have a universe of movement surrounding our limbs, and by means of our limb system we are able to imitate the movements of the world. The head is there to perceive these movements and bring them to rest. Just as perception of the world around is brought about by means of the nervous system, in the same way there are nerves which become aware of the inner processes, the changes of movement and position of the muscles and the associated chemical changes.

The actual process is made clear by the explanation given in the Curative Education Course (30 June 1924*). Here Rudolf Steiner depicts the head and the limbs as two different entities—the one as a metamorphosis of the other.

As already described, the physical organization in the head is located

---

* *Curative Education* (12 lectures for doctors and curative teachers, Dornach, 25 June–7 July 1924).

on the outside, in the bones of the skull; going inwards are the ether, astral and ego organizations. In the digestive-limb system it is the other way round. 'In the metabolism and limb system, on the other hand, the ego is on the outside, vibrating all over the organism in its sensibility to warmth and touch. Proceeding inwards from the ego, we have then the astral body vibrating in an inward direction; farther in it all becomes etheric; and finally, inside the bones it becomes physical.' This explanation clearly shows what it is that mediates between the movements in the surrounding world and the human movements. It is the ego that lives in the warmth around the limbs. It penetrates into the astral body, the ether body and the physical body, and thus movement arises in the limbs.

In the healthy organism the cosmic movements are reflected in a harmonious way, as happens in the artistic form of eurythmy which *then* works as a healing influence on the spectator.

In the patient, disturbances arise in the sick organism which can make the movements distorted, twisted, cramped, frozen, jerky and uncontrolled.

'Curative eurythmy grows out of the movement-gestures of pure art, and of educational eurythmy when they are modified in such a way that they emanate from the unhealthy being of man, as in the first place they spring from the healthy.' [*Fundamentals of Therapy.*]

The task of the curative eurythmist is to be a mediator between the irregular movements of a sick organism and the ideally healthy and healing movements of universal nature; and also to cultivate the sound-gestures as perfectly as possible in one's ether body, so that they work upon the maladjusted movements of the patient. Eurythmy makes the sounds artistically, by means of one's own body. Thus, there is a great difference between the practice of artistic eurythmy and curative eurythmy. For this reason the two should not be combined. The basic principles of both are the same, but the aims are different. Even in the first lecture of the Curative Eurythmy Course Rudolf Steiner says: 'But for those who wish to engage in artistic eurythmy, I must expressly emphasize that they will have to forget entirely what they have learnt here if they want to go on with eurythmy as an art . . . and whoever tries to combine the two will, in the first place, destroy his artistic power, and secondly, he will not be able to achieve very much as regards the therapeutic element in eurythmy.

In the practice of curative eurythmy it is necessary to cultivate the powers of observation. Anything that has to do with movement should be of interest. The growing number of patients suffering from handicaps of movement shows how endangered the movement-system is today. Therefore any therapy undertaken in this field will become of ever-growing importance. New ways are always being sought in movement therapy to treat the various illnesses showing all kinds of symptoms of paralysis and the growing number of brain-damaged children with their hemiplegia and paraplegia, with their hypomotility and hypermotility.

As a result of our civilization, with its techniques of locomotion and its mechanization in industry, the great danger arises that the connection with natural movements will be cut off and our movements will be impoverished and no longer serve as an expression of the inner life. A repetitively executed mechanical movement on a machine can jostle out of existence the movements permeated by our own life of soul and spirit. As the movements and gestures are altered through minding a machine, we see how thinking, feeling and willing come into them less and less. When a craftsman in times gone by made an object, the idea, the image, of the thing he was making flowed into his skilful hands. Since this is becoming less and less the case in the piecemeal manufacturing process of modern industry, we are becoming more and more dull in our movements.

It is even worse when human movements are taken hold of by powers from another world which is emancipated from below nature, introducing man to sub-human forces. Thus movements arise which neither belong to the cosmos, nor are they purely earthly-mechanical ones. This is a sub-natural world of movement, foreign to man. We can observe it in children suffering from damage in the mid-brain. Meaningless, chaotic, unrhythmical movements appear which have no real purpose. No expression of soul flows into them—they serve, in the end, only for destruction. It is for just these movements that curative eurythmy can be of such special significance.

*

If we are going to use eurythmy as therapy, there are two conditions to be fulfilled which are necessary in every therapy:

1   an accurate diagnosis;
2   a systematic treatment aimed at the specific complaint.

We shall see in further detail how curative eurythmy can be applied to these conditions. The particular exercises have a specific effect on certain illnesses. Curative eurythmy is not a vague, indefinite movement-therapy. In the transformation of eurythmy into curative eurythmy Rudolf Steiner has shown how an art can be metamorphosed into an art of healing.

CHAPTER 2
The Alphabet

Since eurythmy is visible speech, it follows that it is bound by the laws of language. Our alphabet contains only a few sounds, yet everything that we want to express—about our inner life, when we want to describe the beauties of the laws of nature, all the results of human research, all poetry—can be done through the combination of these sounds. In earlier times people knew that every sound had its own intrinsic meaning. Each sound had its own name: Aleph, Alpha, Beta ... each revealed something of what lay behind it as divine-spiritual being. Each single sound was experienced as part of the divine creative Word. Mysteries of the world and of the human being could be experienced through meditation and contemplation of sound as such. Language could only sound forth out of the human being because the creative Word was active within him and he learned how to re-create and utter it as speech.

So it was in ancient times. Something of this still comes down to us in Plato's Dialogue 'Kratylos', for instance. Kratylos represents the point of view that everything that has been created—stone, plant and animal—has its own right name, the eternal name, given to it by its own nature and by the creative Word. In the periodical *Natura*, Vol. V, 1928/9, Ita Wegman speaks about Kratylos. As regards eurythmy, it is of particular interest to us that Kratylos attached as great a significance to the gesture as to each sound itself, and perceived reality in both. He experienced each separate sound as gesture. This is made clear in the following quotation from the article mentioned above:

> Kratylos, asked by Socrates about the essence of sound, confirms that in the pressing together of the tongue in 'D–T' there is something binding in the 'D', while something firm and steady is imitated in 'T'. In 'L' is a soft, gliding together with something smooth, oil, gluey. In 'O', on the other hand, there is something round, and 'R' embraces every movement; while 'I' (ee) again expresses as sound-gesture something thin and fine.

In ancient Hebrew times also, there existed a deep knowledge of the alphabet. During the last century Eliphas Levy published the following significant sentences about the first seven sounds of the Hebrew alphabet from a sixteenth-century Hebrew manuscript:

A *Aleph*—he sees God face to face without being overcome by death and speaks confidently with the seven Genii who command the whole heavenly Host.
B *Beth*—he stands above all afflictions and fear.
G *Ghimmel*—he rules with the whole of Heaven, and the whole of Hell serves him.
D *Daleth*—he ordains his own and others' health and life.
H *He*—he is not surprised by any misfortune, nor oppressed in any adversity, nor overcome by any enemy.
V *Van*—he knows the meaning of past, present and future.
Z *Dzain*—he knows the secret of the resurrection of the dead, and possesses the key to immortality.

Every single sound expresses tremendous things about the being of man. This deep wisdom in the sound is now lost to us, but Rudolf Steiner has shown us how to regain this knowledge in a new way. If we look first at the consonants we see that the way in which they are allocated to the lips, teeth and palate indicates the connection with the human organism.

The customary arrangement is to be found in the Curative Eurythmy Course:

Labial sounds: w b p f n r
Dental sounds: d s sh l n r
Palate sounds: g k ch (as in lo*ch*) ng r

It will be noted that r belongs in all categories.

In the lectures on 'Speech and Drama' [5–23 September 1924] Rudolf Steiner goes into still more detail:

1 Labial sounds: m b p
2 Lower lip, upper teeth: f v
3 Teeth together: s tz z
4 Tongue behind upper teeth: l n d t (hard palate)
5 Soft palate or gutteral: g k r y qu

This arrangement points to the threefold nature of man. The labial sounds give an inner compactness to the whole form. If a child habitually has its mouth open, this nearly always shows some abnormality, usually a slow development or even weak-mindedness. If the labial sounds are practised in eurythmy with these children, keeping in mind that the whole organism, including the lips, does the sounds as well, an improvement in the control of the body can soon be seen. If one observes in a patient that the co-ordination is poor between the upper and lower lips, that the movement of the lower lip does not conform to that of the upper lip, it will often be found that there is a predisposition to an illness, especially of the nervous system. The right co-ordination between the lower and upper lips is of great significance for the whole organism.

The dental sounds can serve to bring about a balance between the lower and the upper organization. For instance, 'D' as a sound acts upon the harmonization of the blood circulation and the breathing.

'G', 'K' and the other soft palate sounds lie furthest back in the speech apparatus, deep down in the organism. They are connected with the limbs of man and with the unfolding of the will. Children who can pronounce the soft palate sounds well usually stand firmly on the ground with their feet. We could see the magnitude of these connections in a small patient. The little girl could walk well alone and say all the sounds; then she injured both her heels and had to walk on her toes. After a time she also lost the ability to pronounce the soft palate sounds.

A second arrangement of the consonants leads us in a different way to the human organization:

Explosive sounds: b d g k m n p t
Breath sounds: h v f s sh ch (as in lo*ch*)
Vibrant sound: r
Liquid sound: l

The explosive sounds are formed differently from the breath sounds in eurythmy. With the explosives one tries to present the plasticity of the sound by bringing out the initial movement and then holding on to it for a moment. The breath sounds are performed in a more mobile way. The vibrations of sound-gesture are reproduced with the whole body. With the explosive sounds we 'assert the inner world', while with the breath sounds we are 'carried into the outer world'.

Between explosive and breath sounds we have the liquid sound 'L' and the vibrant sound 'R'. This arrangement of the consonants shows their connection with the elements.

The solid, with the life ether belonging to it, are connected with the firmness of the explosive sounds.

The flowing 'L' lives in the watery element and the chemical ether connected with it.

The air, and with it the light ether, are expressed in the rolling 'R'.

Finally, the warmth and the warmth ether live in the breath sounds as they stream out.

A third differentiation of the consonants is in the colouration through the vowels. When the vowel which accompanies the consonant stands in front of it, e.g. 'el', then the desire to remain inside is stronger, whereas with 'la' or 'ka' there is a direct connection with the outside world. One has to learn to observe whether a person wants to remain more within himself, or whether he easily goes out to the spiritual in the world. In practice one learns to recognize whether the patient is making an 'ek' or a 'ka'. Often the exercise can be made easier if one makes the patient do 'fi' instead of 'ef'. In the musical Italian language many sounds are still tinged with the rhythmical element, e.g. 'ele', 'eme', 'ene'.

*

If we turn now from the consonants (*consonare* = sound with) to the vowels, we find that they are what could be called 'self-sounds', that is, they express experiences of the inner self:

*'A' —I am amazed, I wonder ('A' as in f*a*ther)
'E' —I defend myself ('E' as in *ei*ght, or f*a*te)
'I' —I assert myself ('I' as in m*e*)
'O'—I embrace the world lovingly ('O' as in *o*val)
'U'—I am afraid ('U' as in m*oo*n)

This sequence of vowels pictures the whole development of mankind.

Again, let us consider the alternating vowels and consonants as the letters succeed each other in the alphabet. The firm explosive sounds are followed by the selfless, yielding breath sounds in continual alternation. And from time to time the expression of an inner soul-experience is inserted by means of a 'self-sound'.

'A' stands at the beginning, in the very first place. It is the sound of childhood, the sound of wonder with which every normal child really finds its way into the world. To wonder at, to be amazed at something, is a very real power which is the beginning of all knowledge and understanding.

Man feels himself wrapped in his own sheath, his own house against the world: 'Beta'. In the sound 'C',† he experiences the lifting up of weight. 'Heaviness made light' is what is expressed in 'C'. In 'D', man looks at the world of the senses, lives and breathes with the things around him. Next comes 'E', one of the 'self-sounds': 'The world has done something to me, I defend myself.' One tries to understand oneself in contrast to the world.

We see in the alphabet how explosive and breath sounds continually alternate with one another; and herein lies revealed the wisdom of its composition. For the succession of explosive and breath sounds, the inner control through the 'self-sounds', works right down into each separate organ and gives to each the right configuration. Form and process alternate.

The alphabet begins with the weaker explosives: 'B', 'D', 'G'. They are repeated later, like a reflection, in a stronger form: 'K', 'P', 'T'. A

---

* *Translator's note:* These pronunciations are adhered to throughout.
† The author is here describing the German 'C' which is pronounced 'Ts'.

group like 'H-I-K' is interesting: in 'I' the human being asserts himself in the balance between the strong breath sound 'H' and the strong explosive sound 'K'. Another trio which is used in curative eurythmy is 'L-M-N'. Through 'L' the feeling for life is stimulated and strengthened; through 'M' the forces are brought into the breathing out; and with 'N' they are conducted towards the activity of the head.

It will become clear to us that the alphabet is not an arbitrary collection of sounds, but that it is governed by a deep wisdom. What is it trying to reveal to us? The mysteries of man's evolution that lie hidden in it. The laws of the etheric body weaving and forming its images lie unseen within us. 'When we put the alphabet together from beginning to end (A-Z), a very complicated word arises, but this word contains all the possibilities of word-formation. This word, however, contains at the same time the human being in its etheric nature.'

The alphabet in itself is an exercise in curative eurythmy. If it is performed in front of someone who is very ill, the tranquillizing, beneficient, healing effect becomes apparent.

CHAPTER 3

Practical Application

A few basic principles will be indicated for the practical application of curative eurythmy. As in all therapy there are no hard and fast rules or instructions that can be given. Every patient who comes to curative eurythmy is a new question for us. All expressions of movement should be of interest to us and then the movements—be they well done or not—will show us what the organism needs. The sounds themselves will be our best teachers in therapy. Over and over again we shall have to deepen our experience of the nature of sound; it is an inexhaustible fount.

Before proceeding with a description of individual sounds, some general remarks about all vowels and consonants must be made.

What follows may be taken as the standard method of practising the *vowel* sounds:

1 The vowel is sounded aloud, with the arms held at rest.
2 The sound, e.g. 'A', is formed, beginning high up, then returning to the rest position; the next 'A' is formed a little lower, and again back to the rest position, and so on, until the last 'A' is formed as low as possible (and at the same time as far behind as possible). Now the arms are returned to the 'A' position at the top and swung through all the previously formed 'A' positions (while the arms keep the same angle with which the exercise began). The swinging gets faster and faster and stops when the movement is at its fastest.
3 In quiet concentration we try to hear the sound as we first spoke it aloud, echoing within us.
4 Now we jump into the sound with the legs, moving either forwards or backwards.
5 We repeat the whole arm exercise, i.e. all that was given in 1, 2, and 3 above, once more.

The exercise with the legs should occupy about one third of the total time taken for the whole exercise.

The quiet concentration, listening to the re-echoing of the spoken sound, is of particular importance. Through it the effect of the vowel that was performed is directed upon one's own body and the full therapeutic effect is thereby achieved. An important part is missed if this is not done.

Practical Application

This quietness after the vigorous movement is an important part of the exercise. Some shrink from using it at first, but it is soon found that patients like doing it. This can be carried out even with children, when one adopts this inner attitude of listening oneself; the inner calm and attention has to be conveyed to them by the curative eurythmist. One can practise allowing the sound to re-echo within, either once, after completion of the whole exercise, or each time after doing the arm exercise, i.e. twice.

Turning now to the consonants, the effect on the body of the sound which has been practised is achieved in a different way. We form the consonant, for instance the 'B', in curative eurythmy and at the same time we imagine ourselves in this gesture. We make a picture therefore of ourselves during the exercise, as if we were looking at ourselves in a mirror. This exercise requires imaginative power. If it is repeated often it will be found that the curative effect, also on the patient, is strengthened and that it works correctively.

It is not possible to carry out the exercises in the usual way with many patients, e.g. those who are lame or handicapped. Then the artistic and creative imagination must be brought into play. To begin with, the exercise is done only in front of the patient, or the arms and legs of the patient are moved passively into the eurythmic gestures, and in this way one tries to get him to experience something himself. Of course, the gesture which he does out of his own inner activity is the best. Therefore one should try to coax every possible active movement from a handicapped person, be it with fingers, toes or eyes. To demonstrate the sound in such cases is effective, even when it seems to elicit little response at first. When only one side is paralysed then the movement is done first by the healthy side, and the paralysed side tries to imitate it and finish it—or at least pictures it in the imagination.

Corrections should be avoided as far as possible. During the eurythmy training they are, of course, necessary, but in curative eurythmy one is dealing with sick people who are looking for help, not instruction. The doctor does not blame the patient when a remedy does not have the desired result. He looks for the reason and changes the medicine or gives a stronger dose. So also in curative eurythmy. If a sound cannot be formed well, or the movement cannot be completed or be penetrated sufficiently by the soul, it often helps to let the patient just imitate. It is always important to let the patient be active so that he develops his own connection with the sound and accepts the exercise positively. Then the exercise becomes a joint activity. If one can see where the difficulties lie, one can often help by paying special attention to that part of the body where the movement begins (in the shoulder or wrist, etc.). A picture, a comparison or a well-chosen word will inspire one at the right moment to help further in such cases. One can nearly always rely on co-operation from the patient, since people today like to do movement exercises and to work towards their own recovery.

In children, we have the good fortune to be able to appeal to their powers of imitation. It is always a surprise when a badly handicapped child with but small means of expressing himself imitates an 'A' or a 'U'. With the help of this innate ability it is possible to introduce curative eurythmy to all, even the worst cases. If the ability to imitate is lacking, then we must try to awaken it, for instance, by practising 'A-E-I—I-E-A' (see Chapter 5).

Some special exercise will be dealt with later in the book. There are many ways of dealing with the various cases and it will always be possible to select the right one if you go back to the original indications. In building up a particular treatment it is good to start with some preparatory exercises, such as stepping or rhythms, until the patient gains a certain inner composure. If you have to do a sequence in curative eurythmy, such as 'L-M-R', then you work at each sound separately and always come back again to the whole sequence. Also at the end the whole exercise should be done again.

If it is possible, it is very important to let the patient rest for a longer or shorter period after the curative eurythmy treatment.

It is useful to make changes in the tempo of the exercises. You can start slowly, then get quicker and at the end take it more slowly again. In all the changes of tempo you are appealing to the ego. Some exercises actually specify the acceleration.

*

In curative eurythmy the sound, or sequence of sounds, which has been prescribed therapeutically according to the diagnosis, has to be repeated many times. The whole value of the therapy lies in reinforcing each sound and in the repetition of the same exercise. The same exercise is practised for days, weeks, and sometimes even for years. The actual therapeutic exercises are done until the disturbance has been resolved. Prophylactic exercises or exercises for constitutional disorders often have to be continued for a very long time. In such cases it is good to introduce, in the right way, changes in the exercises—that is, to do one exercise for a few weeks and then take another exercise for a few weeks. It will also be found from experience that interruptions are beneficial. After a period of rest, the results which were aimed at are confirmed and, indeed, often even improved upon. In deciding for how long an exercise should be continued, it will be necessary to consider whether the effect of the exercise is directed more towards the ego, the astral body, the etheric body, or the physical body. In a lecture [21 December 1908], Rudolf Steiner speaks in detail about the rhythms of the various members of our being. Here it will be only briefly mentioned that the ego-rhythm is the 24-hour rhythm, that is, the daily rhythm, as such. The rhythm of the astral body is the seven-day rhythm; that of the etheric body, four times seven days; and that of the physical body is the yearly rhythm (ten times seven times four days in a woman, and twelve times seven times four days in a man). At the beginning of a treatment it is usually best if the patient can come several times a week, or even every day, for the lesson, until he has found his own relationship to his exercises and—as is often possible in many cases—can then practise alone at home and need not come so often for the lesson. Many people find it a great help, long after they have been discharged from treatment, for instance to practise 'I-A-O' in the mornings, or to prepare themselves for sleep in the evenings by doing slow walking, 'A-Veneration' or 'Hallelujah'. It is even sometimes possible for the doctor to show the patient an exercise when he comes for consultation and then let him do it at home, as long as he is kept under frequent observation.

In general a curative eurythmy treatment can last for half an hour, not longer. This is regulated by what the patient is capable of achieving.

In schools it is usually sufficient to practise curative eurythmy just for a short time with the children. According to suggestions given by Rudolf Steiner in the weekly teachers' meetings which he attended at the Waldorf School, 'The child should do curative eurythmy exercises for a certain length of time, and they should be done daily'; and 'If a child is given a curative eurythmy exercise, it is because he is ill. Since this is a therapy, it must be made possible for the child to be fetched out of any lesson.'

If the patient cannot do the exercise every day, then a good rhythm must be found. In our institutions for children in need of special care the following rhythm has proved valuable: Monday, Tuesday, Wednesday and Friday working with the children, while Thursday is a rest day. It is best to choose a time in the daily rhythm which can be adhered to. Sometimes an exercise can be done three times daily, or at intervals of from four to six days, according to instructions. Sleep exercises can very well be done with good effect in the late evening, or immediately before going to bed.

The child should not do artistic eurythmy before he has completed his third year, since until this age cosmic forces are at work in him. But for *curative eurythmy* it is different. If abnormalities appear, e.g. inability to sit or stand up, squinting, deformation of the body, etc., then exercises can be started very early, but of course in a way that suits the child.

Further, it is accepted in eurythmy that pregnant women should not do any sort of eurythmy. It is allowable to do gentle exercises in curative eurythmy during pregnancy if troubles arise, but care should be taken that the abdomen is completely relaxed and at rest. And only those curative eurythmy exercises that are absolutely necessary should be done. There are special exercises given for a tendency towards miscarriage (see Chapter 11). These, however, should only be done between pregnancies. Certain curative eurythmy exercises, like 'M' for menstrual difficulties or 'B' for migraine, should not be done during periods of pain. In cases of bone fracture, where a limb has to be immobilized for a time, it is sometimes of great benefit to practise with the healthy limbs. Curative eurythmy is not advisable during acute illness, with high temperatures, or conditions of extreme exhaustion.

Curative eurythmy can often show good results even after the first few lessons, but sometimes only after weeks and years of quiet perseverance. In some illnesses, for instance paralysis, one has to be content if only the attitude to life has altered, without much external change being apparent, or, in the case of an epileptic, if the fits do not altogether cease but become less severe and occur less often, or his general dullness diminishes.

And now, a word about the health of the curative eurythmist. It is often asked: How many hours a day can one practise with patients or children? Here, too, it is difficult to make general rules. It depends on the individual's strength, and also on the methods employed. Is it not harmful to oneself to do all the different exercises, including the spoken part, with the various patients? These questions are very frequently asked. Gradually one will develop a feeling for what is right for oneself—and also for the patient. One has to show him what to do, and encourage him, and then hold oneself back in order to watch and to allow him to unfold his own activity. Indeed, patients are often very grateful to be left alone for a while, so that they can try it out quietly for themselves. It is important for the practising curative eurythmist to go back again from time to time to artistic eurythmy to be refreshed, and also to avoid becoming one-sided. Another question that one always meets is: Does the curative eurythmist give of her own etheric forces? Curative eurythmy is not a magnetopathic treatment—that is just what is so wonderful about it, that the healing powers are the sounds themselves and we are only the mediator. When curative eurythmy is being done there should always be present: the patient, the curative eurythmist and the healing reality of sound.

CHAPTER 4

The Vowels

We will now speak about the effectiveness of the vowels 'A', 'E', 'I', 'O', 'U'. The diphthongs 'Ei' and 'Au' are not given as curative eurythmy exercises. Starting with the paradigmatic phrases given by Rudolf Steiner for each vowel sound, we shall try to explain the specific range of these sounds which we have gained from experience so far, while always remembering that we are at the very beginning of this new therapy movement and the following issues can therefore only be regarded as indications.

The sound 'A' (ah)

In the sound 'A' we express one of the fundamental feelings of the soul: wonder, astonishment. Even today it is still one of the few primary gestures, to open the arms wide in amazement at something new, thus giving oneself up to it.

'A' is an ensouled gesture which opens at an angle. In curative eurythmy the 'A' is formed, beginning above, high up, and getting lower and lower, while at the same time taking care that the angle remains the same. The main principle underlying the effect of 'A' is:

> 'A' works against the animal nature in man and ... when it is practised very often, then this is the exercise which should be used for people who are *greedy*, in whom the animal nature is particularly strong. If you have a child in the school, for instance, who is like a real little animal in every way, and in whom this characteristic is organically based, and you then let the child do this exercise, you will see that it means a great deal to him ...

In order to understand the physiological effect of 'A', we must look at the twofold nature of the human soul. *One* part of the soul opens itself in wonder at the world; it wants to open itself to the spirit. The gesture for 'A' is an expression of this. Rudolf Steiner has spoken many times about the wonderful things that lie within the sound 'A'. To mention only one:

> The realization that man, as he stands before us as a physical being, is but a

part of the complete human being, and that we only have the real man before us when we perceive the full measure of the divinity within him—this realization, this wonder called up in us by a contemplation of our own being, was called by a primeval humanity: 'A'. 'A' corresponds to man in his highest perfection . . .

The *other* part of the soul is turned towards the animal nature; it tends to become greedy. It is that part of our soul which connects itself with the body, with the actual organs, through which we feel hunger, thirst and all the other cravings. This twofoldness of the soul has been expressed by Goethe in the words spoken by Faust:

> Two souls, alas! reside within my breast.
> And each withdraws from, and repels its brother.
> One with tenacious organs holds in love
> And clinging lust the world in its embraces;
> The other strongly sweeps, this dust above,
> Into the high ancestral spaces.*

It is not easy to imagine how the 'A' is connected with 'two souls'. Rudolf Steiner makes it clear in saying: 'when we say "A" we have a feeling as if something spiritual enters into us which is related to our soul and really divides us into two.' [Elizabeth Baumann.] The activity of the astral body in man carries the signature of twofoldness. Even if it has to be regarded as one whole, its activity is still different in the upper and the lower being of man because of the different ways in which the members of our being interact upon each other. If we picture a lemniscate to ourselves it will make the polaric working clear. In the lower part, the astral body works in the organic activity, in the assimilation, the digestion and the excretion of substance. In the head it is free of this organic activity and promotes perception and thinking. In the lectures *The Evolution of Consciousness* Rudolf Steiner enlarges on the lemniscate as a picture of the twofold soul as follows. In earlier times the upper part was the more active and was larger than the lower part. Because of this larger upper part, higher beings exercised divine influence over man. To attain freedom, however, this influence had to diminish and it was in the year AD 333 that the upper and lower parts became equal. Since then the lower part has been growing larger and therefore humanity is in danger of the soul becoming too strongly bound to the earth and to the organism, and of losing those beings who were connected with its earthly origin.

In the repetition of the 'A'-exercise, the upper, luminous part of the soul is influenced by the ego and strengthened. This strength also

---

* *Faust*: Part 1, Scene 2, Easter Promenade. Bayard Taylor's translation.

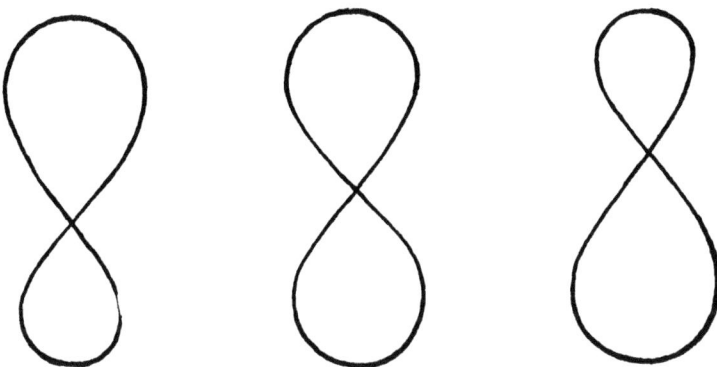

permeates the organic part of the astral body and thus works against the animal nature. Soul and spirit penetrate the bodily organization more fully. In this way 'A' always works in the sense of an incarnating process.

The predominance of the animal nature in man can make its appearance in many different ways. When the child is born he is in a horizontal position to begin with, a position in which the animal always remains. But the child has to overcome this situation and stand upright. He begins by lifting his head and stretching out his little arms and hands. Many of these movements are reminiscent of the 'A'-gesture, and indeed, 'A' is to be seen in the whole bearing of a small child—in the way in which he opens his arms, the first steps with wide-spread legs, yes, even the first wide gaze of the eyes. 'A' is the sound of early childhood. It is also often the first sound which the child utters. It helps the process of incarnation, for the 'A'-movement of grasping the world in two directions has its opposite movement in the influx of the spirit. This incarnation process can be upset; the being of soul and spirit can fail to enter in the right way. The child's body may be formed well enough, legs and arms be well-developed, but they remain flabby and are not capable of making independent movements. The first sign of this is that the child does not raise himself up. He cannot even raise his head without it always falling back again. The child does not try to raise himself in his bed or his play-pen. One feels helpless in this situation and has so little to offer. One can often see miracles happening if 'A' is practised with a child like this. He will almost always enjoy doing an 'A'-gesture if one takes hold of his little arms and helps him do the movement, and much may be achieved if one carries on patiently.

There is another factor connected with standing upright, and that is the involvement of the soul in the sense perceptions, and the wonder at the newly found world around. It is marvellous when a child gradually learns to feel the qualities of warmth, colour and sound in the world around him, and to see his eyes light up. The soul's power of feeling streams into the senses and grasps the world with it. This, too, is achieved through the 'A'-gesture.

In this grasping of the sense-world, greed and desire can get entangled; the lower nature of the passions can become intrusive. It can come to expression in an exaggerated appetite for food, but also in many other ways. For instance, a child wants to have what it sees. There are children who reach for everything: they want to grab all the toys for themselves, only to drop them again the next minute, or even smash them. Much of what our civilization offers the senses appeals to the lustful nature in man and feeds it. Advertising reckons with greed and the instinctive passions, and leads to over-production.

Greed, expressed as movement, is a gesture of pressing forward, rushing forward, head down, and herein lies the danger of losing the upright position. Imagine, beside it, the gesture for 'A'—the upright stance, the controlled restrained power—and it can readily be seen from observation that here is a means of curbing the passionate nature.

The predominance of the animalistic nature is one of the causes of kinetic disturbance in children. They cannot keep their limbs still, but attack everyone and easily become quarrelsome. In one such case 'A' was an important diagnostic factor for me. A 9-year-old boy, who was called a 'nuisance' by his family because of this restlessness, showed, in forming an 'A', that there was a morbid etheric asymmetry between left and right. Physically he was well-formed, but when he did 'A', the left side was completely penetrated, while on the right side the 'A' could not be properly formed; the active permeation of the arm reached only about as far as the elbow. It is understandable that a child does not feel well in these circumstances, since he does not find the inner balance of forces in the etheric, and the asymmetry offers resistance to the penetration of the spirit-and-soul. In this case 'A' helped after only a short period. Similar trouble as described above can also be the underlying cause of St Vitus' dance.

Again, the lower instincts in man can lead to his being overwhelmed by his desires and digestive forces, becoming dull in his thinking and not awake in his sense organs. It can even go as far as migraine, where all sense perception becomes painful and thinking is hindered. For migraine-digestive disturbances we combine 'A' with a consonant as determined from the diagnosis, but especially with 'B'.

'A' is also suggested for over-stimulation of the sexual organs. In this case it should be done with the hands, fingers, knees, toes and eyes.

An 'A'-exercise done in the morning can facilitate the process of waking. But 'A' helps just as much for sleeplessness. In the latter case 'A-Veneration' is primarily used. In this exercise 'A' is done strongly forwards and, while holding the 'A', an 'H'-gesture is made with the shoulders, through which the feeling of veneration is expressed. By doing the 'A' backwards, slowly, we free ourselves from the world of the senses and become submerged in the world lying behind us. If this is practised often the organic powers of resistance will be strengthened. Veneration for something great conquers one's own egoism. It is an exercise which can be counted among the hygienic-prophylactic exercises and may be done unhesitatingly for a long time. It develops devotion in the soul, and in the body makes the organism capable of warding off external influences. It strengthens the inner resistance and can be helpful in every form of allergy. For insomnia it is especially recommended in those cases where the day's impressions and thoughts about the day's events are a hindrance to sleep. In performing the backward movements there should be no stiffening of the neck; the whole object of the exercise is for the etheric to be able to free itself in the head.

'A' is joined to 'H' also in the 'eurythmic laughter' exercise. In this exercise 'H' is performed strongly with the shoulders, followed by 'A'. There was some uncertainty about how the 'A' should be formed in this exercise, and I was able to ask Rudolf Steiner about it. He replied that in *this* exercise the 'A' should always be done downwards. In cases of depression, combined with numbness in the shoulder region, this exercise will ease the breathing and will have a loosening, freeing effect.

*

There is something of importance still to be mentioned: the relationship of 'A' with the kidneys. Only through this connection shall we be able to understand that 'A' activates the inbreathing, while all the other vowels strengthen the outbreathing.

The kidneys are the focal point for the astral body to stream in. Usually we regard the kidneys only as an excretory organ. Rudolf Steiner has pointed out to us the important upbuilding process performed by the kidneys. From them the astral body works upon the excretion of water, activates the inbreathing process, and permeates the watery-etheric organism, right to the periphery, with light and air. The tone of the skin, the light processes in the upper being depend upon what streams out from the kidneys. In what is reflected back from the head the 'A' then develops its plastic, formative forces in the organism. We work with this quality of 'A' when the excretory process is poor, or there is malformation of the kidneys. Also in the exercise for the teeth, 'L-A', we reckon with this impelling power of the 'A' coming from the head.

In epilepsy 'A' is one of the most important exercises. It is not the only sound that is used for his illness. Since epilepsy does not show a uniform set of symptoms in all cases, the curative eurythmy treatment has to be different, often using all the vowels, but in certain cases also a sequence of consonants. What has been given on this subject will be found in the relevant chapters. 'A' and 'E' are almost always used.

Epilepsy is a constitutional illness; the entrance of the being of spirit-and-soul is made difficult through the densification of the etheric–physical nature in one or more organs. We know that the etheric and physical bodies remain bound together during the whole of life, while the ego and astral bodies are released during sleep and return on waking to the physical and etheric. Too great density in the bodily organism hinders the proper reunion. Waking up in the morning is always a fresh process of incarnation. We come in with our ego and astral bodies into the physical body, and at the same time we have to wake up, through our organs, into the world of the senses. It is *through* the physical body, not *in* it, that the ego comes into contact with the earthly conditions, the force of gravity, which it overcomes on awakening properly. In the same way, *through* the physical body, the ego is in direct contact with water, air and warmth.

Moreover, the astral body is connected *through* the etheric body with the surrounding etheric world. It permeates not only our own etheric body, but through it becomes engaged in the laws of the etheric world around us in growth, light, chemistry.

In epilepsy there is one or other organ which resists the entry and penetration through it to the surrounding world. The etheric body and physical body are too closely knit together, with the result that the ego and astral body are held up in that organ, without, at the same time, waking up in the world of the senses. In this condition of the body an epileptic fit can occur, so that through the clonic and tonic spasms an entry may be attempted through that organ. For an epileptic the situation is often easier after a fit, until the organ has built up its resistance again. The fit, as such, should not be looked upon as the actual illness; the trouble lies in the organ which has become hardened or congested. In a way, therefore, epilepsy is a difficult waking-up process. 'A', as the incarnation sound, encourages this process of waking-up in the right way.

The basic curative eurythmy exercise of 'A' should be used in such cases in its strongest form, with very rapid swinging. The exercise can be done strongly and energetically; it accomplishes then what is otherwise done through the epileptic fit, but in a controlled, purposeful and therapeutic manner, and makes it easier to overcome the resistance of the organ.

In several cases of epilepsy Rudolf Steiner gave metamorphoses of the 'A' exercise in order to intensify its strength.

A girl, 15 years old, had measles in her ninth year, and directly afterwards epileptic fits. Her periods started when she was 13 years old, and the fits became more frequent either before or after her period. The patient was big and strong, with a rush of blood to the head. Her soul development did not keep pace with her age—she was slightly infantile. In this case the following 'A' exercise was prescribed: one step forwards with the left or right foot, then first the front knee and then the back knee bent to an 'A' angle, and then both knees at once quickly straightened.

Another patient, 21 years old, suffered from fainting fits, occurring about once a month since her periods had started. Soon she had the first epileptic fit after previous bodily exertion. Vomiting, headaches and a feeling of anxiety at the heart appeared with it. For years she did curative eurythmy exercises and received medical treatment prescribed by Rudolf Steiner. The attacks ceased completely. But the patient always had to take care. In this case the 'A'-exercise was so transformed that the 'A' angle was made with both knees in a jump—but as the jump was made legs and feet were brought together again.

*

The balance exercises given in the Curative Education Course for epilepsy should also be mentioned here. If it is clear that the sense of balance is upset and symptoms of dizziness appear, then to the 'A'-movement you add the balance exercises with dumb-bells. To begin with the dumb-bells are exactly the same weight, and with them you practise 'A' or another sound. The exercises which are usually done with the rod are also very suitable here. The choice of exercises depends on what the child is capable of achieving. After a while a change is made with lighter or heavier dumb-bells and sometimes the left and sometimes the right is made heavier. The legs can also be weighted; for instance, a bandage may be placed round the ankles in which copper plates of different weights can be inserted, so that the weight can be varied. Through this impediment a stronger consciousness is brought into the limbs—the play between heavy and light awakens the power of keeping the balance.

Another form of epilepsy can be the result of a disturbance in the excretory circulation when the attacks are connected with a sensation of nausea. Balance exercises in the watery element by swimming are applicable here. But also the food intake should be carefully watched, especially the digestion of liquids.

The non-integration in the element of air can be ascertained as the result of irregular breathing. All curative eurythmy exercises which have a beneficial influence on the breathing will be used here.

In almost all epileptics the connection with the warmth element is upset. Therefore it is essential that they should be warmly dressed; in fact, so that they always perspire slightly.

This relationship to the various elements should be taken carefully into consideration, otherwise the desired result may not be achieved with the sound that is being practised.

The sound 'E' (as in day, say, etc.)

'"E" establishes the ego in the etheric body.' This statement shows us the great physiological difference between 'A' and 'E'. In 'E' we do not remain in the realm of the soul. The 'E'-gesture ought to reveal to us how the ego-organization works in the etheric body.

'E' is formed by a crossing of the limbs, thereby making a point of contact. The contact leads us to an experience of our own body. The step from 'A' to 'E' is a big one. When we make an 'A' we open ourselves to two dimensions of the universe. In 'E' the arms are crossed and we shut ourselves off from the surrounding world. The feeling arises: 'the world has done something to me'. But by making a gesture of contact with myself I can stand up to it. At a certain point in his development the child has to make the transition from 'A' to 'E', otherwise he remains in a state of submissiveness to the external world without confronting it consciously—and this is the condition of the feeble-minded child. He stands there and gapes at the world, mouth open, and his perceptions are not made consciously—the step from 'A' to 'E' is not accomplished.

The possibility of bringing man's ego into the realm of perception is created by the fact that we have a left and a right side which come together in the plane of symmetry. 'If the human being had not two ears, two eyes, two nostrils, then his ego consciousness really would not exist. He also needs two hands, and when he claps them together and feels one hand against the other then already something of the ego consciousness is there. We do something very similar when we unite what the eyes and ears perceive separately. Through our sense perceptions we always become aware of the world around us from two sides, left and right. And we are the ego beings that we are only because we make these two lines of perception, from left and right, intersect. Without it we should not be ego beings at all. In order to be an ego being we have to make left and right intersect. [Steiner, 21 November 1914.]

With every 'E'-gesture that we do we express our ego experience on the plane of symmetry.

The basic curative eurythmy exercise is supplemented by many other 'E'-exercises. Every touch of the hand on the body is an 'E'. For instance, when I say to a child 'take hold of your left ear with your right hand, touch the end of your nose with your left hand, take hold of your right arm with your left hand', etc., every time it is an 'E'. This is a difficult exercise for children who do not experience themselves properly in their bodies. One learns things which are also diagnostically important. Often children can 'find' their arms and the whole of the upper body quite quickly, while thighs, knees, toes and so on cause them much more trouble. This exercise has the effect of waking up the sleepy children.

We often see how an 'E'-gesture will be made instinctively in self-defence, and at the same time to enable one to face up to external shock. The simple gestures of clapping one's hands together at unexpected news or the holding of one's head with the hands demonstrate this holding of oneself against external shocks. Rudolf Steiner gave the advice to a patient who was fearful of life and had a tendency towards depression to hold her head in the mornings when she woke up, and say to herself: 'I have got hold of myself.' A child of retarded development had an outward squint, could not concentrate and had a habit of always rubbing his hands together. In order to make the child conscious of this movement he was made to do 'E' a great deal, also with the legs, and he was even made to walk 'E'. For a kleptomaniac child the advice was given to walk 'E' as often as possible during the day, on tiptoe.

To take hold of one's own body means to develop skill. Clumsiness is very widespread today—it can be the result of a great variety of causes, from convulsions to lassitude. There is a special 'E'-exercise for this condition. In the so-called 'Dexterity-E', the 'E' is done with the arms accompanied by an 'E'-gesture with the legs. In this exercise the outer ankle-bone has to knock against the other knee. This hurts if it is done properly, but so it should. And in spite of it, the children enjoy doing the exercise if it is accompanied by a good rhythm.

*

The main indication for applying 'E' is organic thinness—'weak people in whom the weakness really comes from within'.

We will now deal with the polarities of thinness, obesity, malnutrition and overfeeding together, as they are all treated with 'E' and 'O' in curative eurythmy.

The divergencies of the human figure towards thinness or fatness are to be seen as a weakness in the inner constitution of the etheric. The etheric body is in itself a moving, fluctuating organism. There are differentiations in its quality. The whole etheric world, of which the human etheric body is a part, is differentiated into four kinds of ether; warmth ether, light ether, chemical ether and life ether. It would take too long here to go into a detailed account of the four ethers, but books on the subject will be found in the Bibliography (page 172). In a healthy person these four kinds of ether interact in an orderly way with one another. Warmth and light ethers flow through the head into the organism. The watery-ethereal part of the head is so organized that it lets the external ether through, just as our eye lets the light through. This applies mainly to the warmth and light ethers, while the chemical and life ethers flow up through the digestive-limb system to the periphery of the skin. Thus as warmth and light ethers stream in from all sides through the head and flow downwards from above through the body, they meet the chemical ether and life ethers streaming upwards from below through the digestive-limb system. But these different kinds of ethers have to be kept apart, so where they meet there is a kind of etheric diaphragm—which should be imagined as being dynamic rather than spatial. The adjustment takes place in the rhythmic interplay of circulation and respiration. It is of the greatest importance for the organism that it should take place in an orderly way.

And these two kinds of ethers meet each other in man who is so organized that his organization reaches its culmination in keeping apart, in an orderly manner, these two kinds of ethers; on the one hand, life ether and chemical ether streaming from below upwards; and on the other hand, warmth ether and light ether streaming from above downwards.

> You see, when the human being is looked at like this, one says: What really is a human being? He is, as far as his physical body goes, an organic being which holds the two kinds of ether apart in the right way, and then allows them to interact again in the right way. The whole human organization is really so constituted as to allow the two kinds of ether to work together in the right way.
>
> Now we are getting nearer to what I said: The human being is organized through and through. It is, of course, obvious that he is inwardly differentiated also as regards water, air and warmth, i.e. he is organized. He is also differentiated as regards the ethers; but here the differentiation is fluctuating; it is going on all the time, a continual working into each other within man of the light and warmth ethers on the one hand, which pushes downwards and outwards to the periphery from above; and of the life and chemical ethers which pushes upwards and inwards, towards the centre, so to speak. The etheric body of man is thereby brought into being ... The

form which here confronts you has to be understood from the point of view of the interaction of the two kinds of etheric force. [12 April 1921.]

Undernourishment, even though there is sufficient food, occurs when the two ethers streaming in from above—light and warmth ethers—go too far into the lower being and impress upon it too much of the shaping qualities of the upper being. You can get overnourishment, fatness, when the chemical and life ethers are not held back in the digestive tract, but extend their activity too far into the upper being. In the first case the head-nerve system is dominant, and so we get the undernourished, over-intellectual, thin type to deal with. A young, very thin patient in the Clinic in Arlesheim consulted Rudolf Steiner and was given therapy to strengthen the lower organism (compresses of burdock root), and 'E' to do in curative eurythmy. Rudolf Steiner said of him: 'His thoughts are continually poisoning him.' There was another patient of 17 who was shockingly thin, and at the same time clearly showed a much exaggerated intellectuality and great obstinacy. Both these symptoms—a certain etheric rigidity which can appear in the soul as pedantry and melancholia, and the poisoning effect on the digestive organs—very often accompany organic thinness. A thin person is trying to pull himself inwardly together too strongly; there is too much of the 'E'-gesture in the organic nervous region.

In the structure of the nerves the 'E'-gesture is organically established. The nerves coming from the left side and the right side of the body cross over and form the pyramidal tract; the optic nerves cross in the optic chiasma. We have two eyes and two ears, but we see and hear *singly* because we make the directions of perception coming from right and left intersect. As a whole human being we are formed symmetrically with a right and a left side. By bringing right and left into contact we experience ourselves—this is how the ego-experience arises. In doing the 'E'-exercise with the limbs we release the 'E'-gesture fixed in the nervous region, and allow the ego activity to work in the fluidity of the etheric.

In children who tend towards thinness it is often necessary to combine 'E' with an 'L'-exercise. Also other combinations of exercises present themselves. We all know the tall, lanky, pale, anaemic children, usually over-sanguine and fidgety. The sustenance flowing upwards from below is not made use of creatively by the upper etheric forces, but is repelled so that full benefit is not derived from the nourishment. For them we combine 'L' and the 'Fidget-iambic' with 'E'. When dealing with thin children who tend towards melancholia, we do the special exercise given for this condition: 'E' done with the arms behind the back, whereby it is necessary to protect the child's soul well and to observe the effect of the exercise carefully and modify it accordingly. In cases of anaemia we add to the 'E'-exercise an in-winding spiral. Going from the circumference to the centre an 'A' is done with the arms going over into an 'E'. Having arrived at the centre, another inward-winding spiral is commenced.

*

Let us now go back once more to the opening sentence: '"E" establishes the ego firmly in the etheric body.' The question must then arise: What happens to the astral body when the ego intervenes directly in the etheric body? The astral body is the mediator between the activity of the ego-organization and the etheric–physical body. Through its activity it makes the organization disposed to receive the ego. You could call it the path-finder for the ego activity in the organs. The astral body directs itself towards both sides; towards the ego on the one side, and towards the physical–etheric on the other. The tendency can always arise for it to contact the etheric organism too strongly or too weakly.

We have a remedy for both cases in 'E', since it regulates the relationship of the astral body to the etheric body from the ego. 'Thus in all cases where it can be said there is either too much or too little activity of the astral organism, it is often possible to do a great deal with "E"-forms, and the repetition of them.' We have already seen how in thin people the astral body develops too little activity in the rest of the organism when it is fixed too firmly in the realm of the senses. When the astral body works too strongly in the digestive processes it produces spasms. In both cases the astral body is not sufficiently controlled by the ego. By doing 'E'-exercises the ego is impressed upon the etheric body, thus releasing the astral body. This gives 'E' its comprehensive effectiveness as a remedy for the relief of fits.

We have already discussed in detail the connection of the sound 'A' with epilepsy, but 'E' has a special part to play here since it is used in the treatment of the actual fit. It is often possible to curtail the attack if an 'E'-gesture is made quickly when the epileptic aura begins and the patient feels an attack coming. Some patients learn to manage this quickly. It is one of the exercises which can be taught in the consulting room. But the whole of the 'E'-exercise should be carried out in the intervals between attacks.

From what has been said it follows that the 'E'-exercise can be employed in the many forms of muscular spasm, from writer's cramp to the spastic paralysis arising from brain damage. In all spasms very much depends on *how* the 'E'-exercise is done. The point of contact, the entry of the ego, can only be achieved by a flowing movement, and not from a cramped position.

'"E" establishes the ego in the etheric body.' It follows from these words that 'E' must also be active in the bloodstream. There are two 'E'-exercises which are effective in this field: 'Love-E' and 'E-on-the-floor'. In the gesture of love a streaming out into the distance is experienced. This sensation can be brought home to the patient if he can feel himself stretched out to the horizon and then slowly lets the movement slide forward—without guiding it too much himself—and then finish the exercise with a strong 'E'-gesture in front of the chest. The warmth is felt directly and this is important where there is a tendency towards heart disease which is connected with any sort of contraction, such as angina pectoris in coronary sclerosis. 'Love-E' can be used as a prophylactic exercise in this ever-increasing illness (Managers' disease). Everyone can easily learn this exercise and do it for himself—indeed, it is done daily by many people who have discovered its beneficial effect. The exercise shows us the flowing outwards on the one hand, and the renewal of strength on the other hand, which are to be found in 'E'—a rhythmic exchange such as we have in the systole and diastole of the heart. Through the warmth at the centre, in the heart, a relaxation is created in the circulation which reaches to the extremities.

The second exercise—'E-on-the-floor'—stimulates the peripheral circulation. We use it for bad circulation, low blood pressure, slow pulse where the heart is weak and flagging—conditions which often show themselves as fatigue after exertion and as a state of exhaustion.

In this exercise we work from the periphery towards the centre. We do an 'E' with the arms and at the same time walk the 'E' on the floor, facing forwards. This can only be done with a partner. Two people stand, one behind the other, and walk, one forwards and the other backwards, so crossing over to the other side and thus making together an 'E-on-the-floor'. The exercise is started slowly, gets faster and faster, and ends up slowly again. This exercise needs courage and determination because it is done without looking and one person is always moving backwards; it also takes a great deal of concentration to form the cross properly without bumping into each other. With this exercise the circulation is stimulated in the whole organism, in arms and legs, and thus the action of the heart is strengthened.

In the digestive system the point of access for the 'E' is through the gall-bladder. The gall-bladder is closely connected with the liver and is formed by the forces of the planet Mars which is also the source of the 'E' strength (see Chapter 7). The bile pours into the duodenum and together with the pancreatic juice breaks down the food substance almost to the mineral stage, i.e. it is so far destroyed that it loses all its own vitality and chemical properties. This applies especially to fats and proteins. The bile wards off the influences coming from outside in the same way as we have seen the 'E'-process in the nerves resist the sense perceptions. The bile is reabsorbed in the intestines by the blood and is used again in the production of bile. Thus it has its own circulation. It is related through its pigmentation to the blood and iron process. Bile always penetrates the blood completely and is therefore the physical foundation for vigorous activity. When the bile does not function properly, even when the gall-bladder itself is deformed, we can use 'E' in conjunction with other remedies. If the food is not completely broken down by the bile it cannot be fully utilized—the whole digestion suffers and also the formation of blood, and again we have weak, thin people with a tendency to anaemia.

Again and again we have to remind ourselves that through 'E' the ego establishes itself in the *etheric* body, not in the physical body. The etheric body is not subject to the laws of gravity, but to those of buoyancy. 'E' as practised in curative eurythmy can, therefore, loosen an 'E' which has become organically too strongly fixed in the nervous system—it can develop its activity in the circulating blood—relieve tensions between the astral body and the etheric body, and finally it can bring about a right relationship between the etheric body and the physical body. An etheric body which has become too large is made to conform again to the physical body through the ego while an etheric body which is too strongly attached to the physical body is restored to forces of buoyancy. Thus, 'E' controls the relationship between gravity and levity.

We can also draw attention to the following effect of 'E': our brain exists, likewise, in buoyancy. If it were to rest with its full weight of 1,500 grams on the base of the brain, all the vessels there would be crushed. But it floats in the cerebrospinal fluid and thereby loses weight, so that it presses upon the base of the brain with only 20 grams. Also the 4-5 million red corpuscles which are suspended in the liquid of our blood lose as much weight as the fluid which they displace and, therefore, retain only a little actual weight. This relationship between lightness and weight is important for our ego activity. Our power of imagination could not develop in weight, only in buoyancy. On the other hand the 20 grams which the brain weighs have to be penetrated by the ego, otherwise mediumistic, abnormal tendencies can arise. So our red corpuscles have to be held in buoyancy; for with our soul forces we must not succumb to gravity. On the other hand, though, there has to be some weight so that the ego can feel its resistance. 'E' is active in the balance between the forces of buoyancy and gravity, since it has the power to hold the ego firmly in the *etheric* body.

The sound 'I' (ee)

It is said in the Curative Eurythmy Course: '"I" reveals the human being as personality'; also, 'It can be said this curative "I"-exercise is specially helpful for people who cannot walk properly.'

These two sentences direct our attention to walking in the general sense. A person's individuality is expressed in the way he walks. One need only fall in with another person's steps, to imitate his walk, to learn a great deal about him. The timid, tripping gait, the long, swinging stride, whether dancing along on the toes, or setting the heels down firmly on the ground, are all an expression of the personality and how it comes to grips with the world. In walking we are always in an unstable state of balance, i.e. every moment we have to find the balance between right and left, front and back, above and below. It is the ego which holds the balance between these polarities in walking. With each step it has to be found anew. This balance in walking is often upset through illness. An inhibited gait which does not go forward properly is often a sign of nervousness. We see this in shy, and also in depressive people. When the astral body presses forwards eagerly, wanting to follow up the sense impressions, it leads to an over-hasty gait and stumbling over one's own feet, whereby the head is going too fast for the rest of the body. This is described in paralysis agitans (Parkinsonism) as a symptom of propulsion (see Chapter 12).

The balance between left and right is disturbed when the ego forces are weak from illness or exhaustion, or even from alcoholism which, as is well-known, leads to a weakening of the ego-organization in the organic system.

The disturbance of balance between above and below can be clearly seen in manic or depressive conditions. What a difference between the nimble, tripping step of elation and the heavy, dragging gait of a depressed person who can hardly lift his foot from the ground!

The way in which a person walks can reveal his constitution even more intimately if we separate the step eurythmically into its three phases of lift, carry, place. In lifting the will is revealed, in carrying the thought and in placing the purposeful deed. In ordinary walking the three phases merge into one another. In cases of illness one or other of the phases is often upset. Threefold walking is discussed in greater detail in the chapter on hygienic eurythmy (see Chapter 6).

'The 'I'-gesture, which is an assertion of the personality, is expressed by straightening the whole body, including the arms and legs. For the curative eurythmy 'I' it is best to stretch the arms so that the right arm is stretched forwards and upwards, while the left arm is stretched out behind and downwards. Also this is the best position for starting the swinging movement.

The path leading inwards goes from 'A' to 'E' to 'I'. We form 'I' out of the centre of our being, stretching outwards in all directions, and radiating light and warmth. With this the movement now begins to go from within outwards again. The personality, standing in three-dimensional space, has to maintain itself actively therein.

The spinal column is an important expression of the ego-endowed personality. It is not a part of the parallel formation of the skeleton (see 'U'), but is unique. It springs from the pelvic girdle in a free double swing, forwards and backwards, carrying the head poised in balance. It is, indeed, a wonderful column! The spine shows how it adapts itself to the three dimensions of space by the way in which the vertebrae are articulated in the three separate planes. In the thoracic region the successive vertebrae articulate in the forwards–backwards plane. In the neck region a gradual change in the surfaces of articulation, to the up–down plane is achieved, most obviously in the special vertebrae atlas and axis. Descending to the lumbar region we notice the plane of articulation change to the right–left plane. In the free movement of walking the balance of polarities can be found, but only through the spiritual power of the ego can this balanced interplay be achieved. From what has been said in these studies it will be clear that the curative eurythmy 'I'-exercise is the leading one to use for all spinal defects. It should be used in all cases of spinal curvature, kyphosis, scoliosis; whether they are curvatures from front to back, or left to right, the 'I'-exercise is always suitable. But great care should be taken in practising this exercise in all cases of spinal deformity. The 'I'-exercise should never be done without first making sure how it can be safely practised without making the tendency towards abnormality worse. It is often necessary to consult the orthopaedic surgeon. But the 'I'-exercise remains the leading one amongst all the other orthopaedic and gymnastic measures, for through it we strengthen the power of the ego which directs the spinal column.

Rudolf Steiner gave a special combination of exercises for scoliosis: the 'I' is formed with the shoulders held stiffly at the same height. Then a jump is made, either forwards or backwards, into the 'I' position with the feet together. But first an 'L' is made, which is formed in a special way. It is begun by holding the hands together in front of the breast-bone, then making a forward movement in an unfolding gesture. Through the 'L' an attempt is made to loosen what is already too hard and then through the 'I' to re-form it in the right way.

There are always other exercises to be done in addition. Whenever the front–back direction is in disorder, walking backwards consciously, e.g.

in the 'ego-line'—this is discussed in more detail in Chapter 7—can be of great benefit. Concentration exercises have a disciplinary and strengthening effect on the ego, as well as all variations in tempo. It is always possible to compose different combinations of exercises.

In cases of faulty posture caused by torsion scoliosis, steady walking in all directions is to be recommended. Apollonian forms, in which lots of verbs—of duration, active and passive—have to be done, are appropriate; also geometric forms pointing in all directions of space, e.g. the pentagram.

In disorders between above and below one has to try to create a balance between heaviness and lightness. When the heaviness becomes too oppressive and one gets tired quickly from standing, this can easily lead to pain in the spine and to disc lesions. It is just the light and free play of these discs between the vertebrae that give the spine its great mobility and suppleness. One of the causes of disc lesions is that the ego-organization is not strong enough to transform the burden of weight into lightness. Therefore, any 'I'-exercise is suitable for the prevention of disc lesions. But if the condition has already set in, then 'I' has to be combined with other exercises. In practice it has proved valuable in cases of disc lesions in the lumbar region to combine the 'I'-exercise with the consonants 'Ts' and 'D'; where the disc lesions are in the dorsal region, with 'L' and 'M'. By means of 'Ts–D' the play of the spine is taken hold of as it alternates between heavy and light, while through 'L–M' the play is between forwards and backwards.

*

Every 'I'-exercise has to be done with pleasure. In this case it is a condition which does not apply to other sounds in the same way. Since with 'I' we encroach upon the expression of the personality, of the self, it must not be done under pressure, but everyone has to want to do it, and do it gladly. So therefore one has to be specially inventive when the 'I' has to be done in cases of illness. Often other exercises which also strengthen the ego by means of balancing opposites must be taken first, before going over to the 'I' itself. Changing rhythms and forms, 'Sympathy' and 'Antipathy', 'Major and Minor', 'Contraction and Expansion', 'Yes and No', are all exercises which, through the transition from one extreme to the other, demand ego activity. With children, ball games may be played where the rhythm of give and take comes in; also ring-throwing where small rings are thrown and caught with outstretched arm. Musical pitch, volume and beat exercises work harmonizingly on the up-down, right-left, back-front directions. Also balancing exercises with dumb-bells belong here, as we discussed in the description of epilepsy.

*

A deficiency of the ego forces is also the underlying cause of all asymmetry in the organism and therefore, here too, we use the 'I'-exercise. Squinting is an asymmetry of the eyes. An inward squint is treated with 'I' done with arms and hands, legs and feet, with special emphasis on the little finger and the little toe. The stretching has to be done very well and this often requires long training, especially for the little toe. In all eye exercises the eyes must not follow the movement, nor should spectacles be worn while the exercise is being done. In performing 'I' for an outward squint the emphasis is laid on the forefinger and big toe. If corrections to the eyes have already been carried out by means of surgery or the wearing of spectacles, it does not mean that the more subtle irregularities have been removed and it is still important that 'I' should be practised. Of course, it is necessary to form a picture of the whole condition of the eyes, since squinting is often combined with long or short sight or astigmatism. Also the feet should always be closely observed. If, besides practising 'I' with the toes, an attempt is made to set the whole foot right—heel, arch, and indeed, walking generally—then an improvement can be hoped for in the eyes as well.

Right-handedness is a physiological asymmetry in a healthy sense. Through the use of the right side, the centre of speech is developed in the left side of the brain and vice versa. This is a fact that clearly shows how movements affect the development of the brain. Rudolf Steiner spoke repeatedly in the teachers' meetings at the Waldorf School about left-handedness and also about ambidexterity. For example, in one meeting in Stuttgart he says: 'She [it was a girl] should be told that she is allowed to use only the right hand for writing. You could try to make her double up her left leg in a crouching position and then jump on the right leg. This child is ambidextrous. In cases of definite left-handedness a decision has to be made. One is able to observe in left-handed people that the left hand looks like the right hand. It could also be tackled by means of the eyes. You let her look at her right arm and let the focus travel down to the hand and back again, and then stretch the arm out. This is repeated three times.'

Another remark about the control of left-handedness says that the right arm should be flung upwards and outwards as if throwing, and also the right leg flung upwards and outwards while, at the same time, hopping on the left leg, 'in order to drive the astral body out of these limbs which it is blocking'. Also alliteration, stressed with the right arm and leg, is given for the control of left-handedness. One should always try to accustom left-handed children to right-handedness while they are still young. The following will show why this should be attempted:

The fact of left-handedness is definitely a karmic one, and in regard to Karma it is a phenomenon of karmic weakness. To take an example: a person who has overworked himself in the previous life, not physically, but altogether, either intellectually or in his emotional life, embarks upon the following life with a definite weakness; he is not able to overcome this karmic weakness in his lower being. That part of the human being which comes from the life between death and a new birth is concentrated in the lower being, while the part which comes from the previous life is concentrated more in the head. What is usually strongly developed is weak, and therefore, the left leg and the left hand are specially engaged as substitutes and have to be used instead. The dominance of the left hand leads to the right side of the brain having to cope with the speech instead of the left side. If this is given way to, a weakness remains for the following (third) earthly life. If one doesn't give in, then the weakness is counter-balanced. [Conference report.]

Only if the changeover from left to right proves harmful should it not be carried out, which, however, will only be in a very few cases. It can happen, for instance, that during the transitional period the ideas can become somewhat scattered, so that 'the child, because it is thinking too quickly, is continually stumbling over its own thoughts'. [Konferenzbericht] Of course it is necessary then to make close observations, and to come to a decision as to whether or not to continue with the changeover. A change from left to right-handedness should not be commenced after the ninth year.

Rudolf Steiner gave a particular warning against the opinion spreading among certain educational movements that it is a good thing to teach children to use both hands equally well and achieve so-called ambidexterity. He said that it could lead to a kind of feeble-mindedness in later life. This is connected with the fact that the human being is not built symmetrically as regards certain organs. In our materialistic age where the human being is so firmly rooted in his organs with his soul–spirit organization, this training for ambidexterity can lead to an inner revolt which results in idiocy. This applies especially to anything that has to be done with the intellect. It does not apply to drawing, for instance, which may safely be done with either hand. Sometimes in the future it may be possible for human beings to make use of both sides without danger, when they are no longer so closely bound up with their own bodily substance. This can only be when the personality, as a spiritual being, masters the body, through warmth, right into the physical. In order to get a better understanding of this a few sentences spoken by Rudolf Steiner are quoted here:

> For you see, that phantom which today figures in ordinary science as the human being, that illusory image which is treated as if it were a chemical configuration, does not exist in reality at all as a live human being. A human being is organized in the fluid element just as in the solid, also in his airy

nature, but especially in the warmth element. And as you come up to the warmth there you find the transition to soul-spirit; for in the warmth you have already the transition from space to time. And it is there that the soul merges with the temporal. By way of warmth you come more and more out of the spatial into the temporal, until, by the various means I have mentioned, it becomes possible to seek morality in the physical. [*Man, Hieroglyph of the Universe.*]

All deformities and malformations are a great hindrance to the unfolding of the individuality in the body. This applies not only to the development of intellectual thought, but also to the development of morality. Today, through the potential of encephalography the large extent to which moral disturbances originate in abnormal brain formation is known. In the Clinical-Therapeutic Institute in Arlesheim, Rudolf Steiner saw a boy with a tendency to cruelty. He pointed out that this was a case of malformation of the occipital lobe, the convolutions of which, in this boy, were not properly arranged, but had formed protuberances and did not cover the cerebellum. Co-ordinated movement and mirror-picture drawing were prescribed for this child. It is the case 'that here the astral body is retarded at the back of the head and the occipital lobes which enclose the lesser brain are stunted and at the same time have swellings. They have only developed materially and have not formed the convolutions sufficiently.' Curative eurythmy and mirror-picture drawing were prescribed as the main therapy for this child. Here are some examples of mirror-picture drawing:

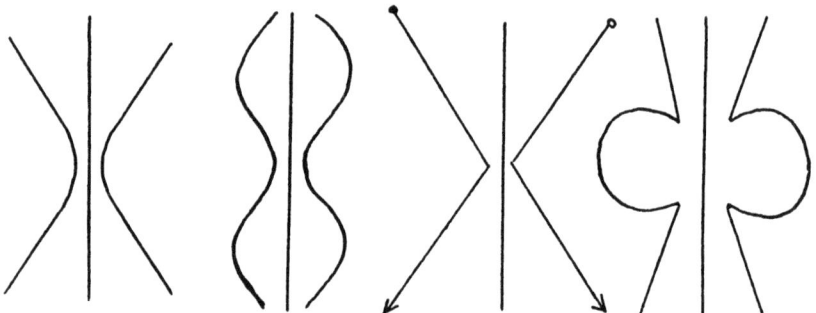

Forms are run in the same way and the sounds made. First one side and then the other is carried out—with arms and legs.

This suggested treatment is not only important for this particular case: we can see here a way that could be significant for all juvenile delinquency. Having established the spiritual facts in this boy's case, Rudolf Steiner went on to say: 'That is the spot where the propensity for cruelty is prevented. A human being has all the instincts within him, but also all the necessary restraints, and they have their localization.' If one turns to a lecture given on 3 March 1916, one finds there too an indication that in all criminal tendencies there is a defective development to be found in the occipital lobe. Thus it is a question of developing the etheric back of the head in such people as early as possible. In youth there is sometimes a chance in this way to change criminal tendencies and even to turn them into a strong and high moral sense.

These co-ordinated movements are to be regarded as ego-exercises and are often done in conjunction with the sound 'I'. Rudolf Steiner gave these co-ordinated exercises to several children in the Waldorf School, e.g. to ones with small heads. Good results were achieved. Even if physically the complete formation of the brain is not attained, nevertheless one is working in a healing way towards creating symmetry in the etheric brain.

In curative education mirror-picture drawing has been developed through many years of practice to a high degree, notably by Hermann Kirchner (Curative Institute, Hepsisau), so that now it has reached its full therapeutic significance for children who are in moral danger.

The co-ordinated movements are equally important when one side is paralysed. The 'I'-movement—or other vowels—are done at first with the healthy side and the affected side completes the movement. If this is physically impossible, then to begin with it can be done in the imagination. Since the etheric is stimulated through the movement of the healthy side, it is often possible, after long practice, for the sick side to join in making the movement. Further details about co-ordinated movements are to be found in *Eurythmy Therapy in Practice* by Elizabeth Baumann.

*

We make use of the correct intervention of the ego to influence processes which cannot start and cannot stop, e.g. in menstruation which is often delayed and then goes on too long. Here 'I', in conjunction with 'M' or 'S', works both on the regulation of the commencement, as also on the proper termination.

For the same reason we do 'I' when the rhythms of evacuation are upset, by involuntary discharge of the bladder and by bed-wetting—but then in conjunction with 'F' and other sounds.

Also in diabetes we use 'I'. Diabetes is an illness in which there is a weakening of ego activity in the digestion. The sugar substance is not broken down sufficiently. And therefore we recommend doing 'I' together with 'D' and 'T', in order to strengthen the digestion in the pancreas and gall-gladder. 'F' can also be used here with good effect.

In the chapter on 'U' we shall describe in detail how the ego-organization has created its pictorial impression of the spirit-soul in the skeleton, and how the skeleton also is moved by the ego-organization.

Next we must consider still another eminent domain of the ego in the human being—the blood. The ego is directly active in the blood, and above all in the warmth of the blood. The ego creates in the blood a balance between the influences flowing into a person from outside through the sense organs of the head and the inner impressions rising up from the various organs within. Here, as everywhere, the ego creates a balance between opposites—spiritually, psychologically, organically and also as a 'mineralizer'. The process of balancing what is unequal is bound up with the substance of phosphorus. Phosphorus is released through the beating of the ego against the red blood corpuscles. We can regard the sum total of red blood corpuscles, swimming about in the lymphatic fluid of the blood, but held in suspension through their iron content, as a mineral boundary wall against which the ego beats.

> What the ego does, is to beat against the blood corpuscles—they are not really globules, but they are intrinsically so constituted that even in their form they show that they are intended to turn movement into equilibrium—which the ego does as it enters into the ability of the human organism to move—including, for instance, the inner movement of warmth. This ego activity reaches its limit in the blood corpuscles and here it has to be intercepted; here must take place that most intimate interchange between the human ego and the whole human organism. [15 April 1921.]

In the watery etheric element 'I' brings about the proper circulation of the blood between the periphery and the centre. In the air-organism again, it is 'I' which plays a leading part in the correct accomplishment of the conversion from breathing-in to breathing-out. Expressed in eurythmy this means that with 'A–E–I' we go inwards from outside, and with 'I' we have the turning point and go from 'I' through 'O' and 'U' to the outside again. In the breath, 'I' connects what happens in the blood and in our inner organs with the environment. Mercurial power is inherent in 'I'. And it is this power which has formed the lungs as an organ, in which the change in the breath takes place, the harmonization between outer and inner; here the rhythms of heart and lungs meet. When this encounter is upset—'I' brings about harmony—it is this aspect that underlies the exercise for stammering.

The deeper one goes into the ideal 'I' and into Rudolf Steiner's words which we quoted at the beginning of the chapter, the more opportunities we shall find for using 'I'. The sound 'I' which reveals the human being as a personality has, understandably, the widest terms of reference.

The sound 'O'

' "O" reveals man as a soul being.' In its effect 'O' is the opposite of 'E'. In 'A' and 'U' we have the polarity between above and below, and can use both to influence growth in these directions. 'E' and 'O' are formed symmetrically bilateral, and influence the tendency to either thinness or fatness. In 'E' we make the right and left sides cross and arrive at an experience of our own selves. In 'O' we form a harmonious circle out of left and right. It is an embracing gesture which brings us a loving experience of the outer world. It is important in the curative eurythmy 'O' that it should be formed equally by both arms, so that from the beginning the roundness is felt all over. Inequalities between right and left often appear in children; one little arm hangs down or cannot come forward quite enough. When this is the case one should take care that no psychopathic tendencies are present. It has been found that this is often so. Pathological children have great difficulty in forming a nice even roundness with both arms at the same height and bringing the fingertips together. When this can be successfully overcome, much has been achieved.

'O' is used therapeutically when there is a tendency to become overweight. If obese people are made to do 'O' one can draw the conclusion that when the inclination towards roundness, which is too strong in the body, is done consciously with the arms, then the tendency is transferred to another plane and this works against the rotundity of the body. The image is strengthened by the manner in which the exercise is done. The patient must imagine, while he is doing the 'O'-exercise, that he has a line drawn against his breastbone, that is, he feels as if he has a spine in front of him which makes the mirror-picture of himself complete at the back. 'O' is accompanied by the 'O'-jump. When this is repeated many times it is extremely strenuous and should never be allowed to go so far as to lead to perspiration.

In the study of the sound 'E' we spoke about the physiological basis for fatness. Only in the right working together of the two kinds of ether, from above and below, can the normal human figure be maintained. We find the reason for undernourishment in the fact that the head forces penetrate too deeply into the lower being. In overnourishment, that which should be worked on by the digestion penetrates too far up into the head. Too much chemical activity and too much life are pouring into the upper part of the being. This has the general effect of blurring and softening the form. The spirit and soul have different functions in the lower and upper part of the human being. Deep down in substance, they activate digestion, growth and upbuilding of the material; while in the soul the will is unfolding. When they are raised out of the material into the upper being they work according to the shape of the head, giving form and shape to everything that is rounded—like the heads of the bones at the joints, and all the surfaces of the organs; in the soul they give form to the thoughts. There has to be a continual rhythmic exchange between above and below which takes place through inbreathing and outbreathing.

'O' lifts the soul out of the material, whereby its formative forces become free so that they can work on the form and shape of the body.

When one gets fat, fat as a substance is deposited. Actually, fat should be entirely consumed by the inner warmth; it does not serve, as protein does, the building-up of our inner structure; it is there for the active organization, to give warmth for movement. The deposit of fat only serves as a padding. Fatty deposits in the body hinder movement, rather than otherwise; they can make one less mobile, both physically and mentally. For since these deposits alter the human form, so also a greater indifference appears in the soul towards this form. It makes one phlegmatic towards one's own feelings. 'If a certain phlegma towards one's own feelings is added to these feelings, then this latter feeling is the result of experiencing the fatty substance in the physical body.' [21 March 1913.]

Physically, an organism that does not use up the fat to produce warmth, but stores it up, will create separate centres of warmth and thus cause a tendency towards inflammatory conditions.

The forces which lead to the storing of fat are animal-astral forces. Indeed they are intensified through storing too much fat in the organs, so that the desire for food grows. If, then, we do 'O' out of our own ego, we subdue the animal-astral forces by raising the soul into its own sphere of light. It will be found that the patient soon benefits from the improvement in the formative forces, that he gains greater control of the organism, perhaps even before there is any noticeable loss of weight.

In order that the soul can really be lifted up out of the organism, the 'O' has to be properly formed. The formation of the ribs and their structure can be an example to us of how the 'O' is organically formed in the ribs themselves. The articulation of the ribs with the spinal column is such that it gives rise to the wonderful curve, and to the rise and fall of the ribs. The head and neck of the ribs lie at the same level as the body and neural arch of the vertebrae—going, at first, from the back towards the front before the forward curve begins. The ribs, too, start with a backward curve before they swing forwards. We begin 'O' also with an upward and backward movement of the arms and only then finish it off with an encircling movement forwards.

It is a known fact—proved by the experience gained from curative eurythmy—that constitutional fatness, as also thinness, is very difficult to influence, since it is something brought from the life before birth. It is influenced by the way in which a person thought in a previous life. Superficial thinking, that only sees things more on the surface, can lead to obesity in this life. It is therefore important to recognize the constitutional disposition early in life and to overcome in children the tendency towards fatness or thinness in later life.

Rudolf Steiner gave some advice which can help in solving this difficult problem. He pointed out that people who tend to become thin in later life are often stiff and inflexible as children, that they have difficulty in bringing out the abilities they have within them. On the other hand, children in whom the watery element predominates and whose physical body is too soft, are inclined to become plump. It will be found that they tend rather to be precocious, and what lives in the mind and soul comes more to the fore.

The child with a tendency to fatness will grasp everything quickly, but he will remain on the surface of things and have difficulty in digesting them; he will not like to do his lessons and does not really quite master them. Organically this means that the spiritual-soul forces are used up by all this brilliance and therefore the organs are not properly permeated. Such a child also lives more strongly in the process of inbreathing than in that of outbreathing. Also he gets easily upset in the air-organism—flatulence, bad digestion, dysfunction of the liver, sometimes at an early age.

As all the vowels, 'O' affects exhalation, but in particular it regulates both breathing-in and out. Its effect can be intensified with the exercise 'O-on-the-floor'. This requires two people, one standing behind the other, in the middle of the room. The one standing behind begins to run in a semi-circle, doing, at the same time, an 'O' with his arms. As soon as he reaches the one in front, this one takes over the movement, and it must always be started by one and taken over by the other. Both together create the form of a circle. The movement starts slowly, gets faster and faster and finishes up slowly again. This exercise often presents difficulty; the circle becomes an ellipse, or it gets corners, and it takes artistic integrity to persevere until a good circle is produced, even when running quickly. Consideration for each other in making one form together is necessary here too, as in 'E-on-the-floor'. This exercise can also be done by fat people as an intensification of the 'O'-effect. It serves to strengthen the diaphragm. Indications for the use of this exercise are diaphragmatic spasms, a tendency to asthma, not breathing deeply enough.

The effect of 'O' on the breathing shows its connection with the air organism. In the exercise for flatulence also, 'L-M-O', and in the one in which 'O' is combined with 'S', we are working on the air organism.

When we go from 'A' through 'E' to 'I' we are going from the outside to the inside. In 'I' we see the turning-point where we start to go outwards again. In the formation of 'O' the power of the 'I' has to work in the organism—only then is it possible to be raised up out of the bondage of the organs.

In 'E' the human being experiences himself—in 'O' he experiences other beings and things. 'A' and 'E' lead towards incarnation, while with 'O' the excarnating process begins: 'In "O" we have the movement whereby the world experiences something through man.'

The sound 'U' (oo)

'"U" reveals man as a human being.' 'U' is used when people cannot stand properly. The upright stature, standing on the earth, shows us the human being as man, and whereby we differentiate him from all other beings in the world.

We form 'U' with a parallel movement of both arms. The curative eurythmy 'U' is intensified by laying the hands together, either with the palms or the backs of the hands; the feet and legs are placed together so that it is almost as if the person were standing to attention. The movement has to be felt through and through. When the arms are stretched upwards the gesture also implies the expression 'I am on the path to the spirit, to myself'—yearning towards union with one's spiritual origin.

We get a feeling of steadfastness from doing 'U' with legs and feet. The feet rest on the ground, ball and heel bearing the weight equally, elasticity in the legs feeling the parallelism up to the hips. The whole figure is sharply defined. The parallel arrangement of the human form is made possible through the shoulders in the upper limbs, and through the pelvic girdle in the lower limbs.

Through 'U' this archetypal picture of the upright human figure can really live in us. Out of this knowledge a wide area of application immediately suggests itself to us. How few of us today really stand properly! To be able to stand still with arms and legs at rest, to stand for any length of time without tiring or getting dizzy, or even fainting, to stand on tiptoe, or on the heels, to stand in the upright position which enables us to listen with even greater mental awareness—all these things are part of being able to stand properly.

Irregularities of posture and collapse of the upright human stature are alarmingly on the increase. In the lower being we see knock-knees, bow-legs, splay feet and flat feet; in the upper being drooping shoulders, a twisted posture and forward stoop. It is all a deviation from the ideal parallelism. Even when there is no visible fault, it is becoming more and more difficult for children to stand still. They continually shift their weight about, fidget, push one hip out, and so forth.

There is now ample experience to show the 'U'-exercise works remedially on all postural faults: on knock-knees and bow legs, on flat and splayed feet. With very small children it is often possible to achieve correction in quite a short time. In the Waldorf School in Stuttgart, even only a few years after its inception, it was confirmed that there were far fewer defects in comparison with other schools. One knows how much trouble and annoyance is caused by continually having to correct children about their posture. Even gymnastic exercises do not always help; nor are supports and bandages, etc. a satisfactory solution for feet that are still growing.

Now let us suppose that with the sound 'U' a very real strength flows into the child again and again, a power which maintains the human being in his given form. Where does this strength come from? Let us go back to the words ' "U" reveals man as a human being.' The human figure is largely determined by the bony system. The hard mineral bones make it possible for man to stand on the earth. In the embryo and during the first years of childhood our bones are not hard; the hard structure is only gradually developed. The ego-organization is active in the formation of the bones. Mineral substances, such as lime, silica, phosphorus, etc. have to be deposited in the other substances which build up the organism, especially in the protein, in order to make the hard bones. It is the ego-organization that is at work here in the deposition of the mineral. The ego is active in the warmth, and cooling-off is also part of the warmth processes. As the warmth diminishes, so the mineral substances are deposited and the bone substance is formed. The skeleton is created out of ego activity and is a physical image of the ego-organization. Thus it can serve the ego-organization for earthly movements. But this is now no longer an inner event, but something that comes from outside.

What Rudolf Steiner has said in the course *Eurythmy as Visible Speech* about the sound 'U' thus becomes clear to us. ' "U" can be felt as something which inwardly chills the soul, so that it takes on a certain rigidity and numbness. That is the inward experience lying behind "U". "U" is the expression of something which chills, stiffens, benumbs and makes one feel cold. "U", then, is the chilling, stiffening process.' This is what the 'U'-gesture shows us. The ego-organization needs this experience to form and maintain the hard bones.

Malformations occur when the structure is not strong enough, and we get troubles such as rickets, knock-knees and bow legs.

The astral body prepares the organs so that they can absorb mineral substance into themselves, but the correct precipitation can only take place when the mineral substance is first brought into the warmth condition so that the ego-organization can work upon it. If the ego-organization is weak, then the precipitation cannot proceed in the right way and rickets and other forms of softening of the bones can occur, as mentioned above. It can also happen that when the ego-organization is weak, the astral body takes over the ego activity. This happens in elderly people when the ego withdraws too soon from the organic activity, but the astral body does not withdraw at the same rate and the dying away process is taken over too strongly by the astral body. Mineral substances then make their appearance in the wrong place and give rise to arterial sclerosis, for instance. This brings us, then, to use 'U' also in cases of senile sclerosis. We must, however, be careful with it. Since the ego is already weakened and the astral body has become too independent as it dies away, one has to use exercises, to begin with, which strengthen the ego and make the astral body pliable again through the ego. Walking backwards, ego-line, 'I'-exercise, in short, everything which strengthens the ego, we combine with 'A-Veneration', with 'M', 'L-M' and 'R'—always with the end in view of getting to the 'U'-exercise at the right moment. Even the first symptoms of arterial sclerosis, such as dizziness and loss of memory, are indicative of 'U'.

The bony system is necessary as a foundation for the human figure, but it is only a foundation. In sleep, or after death, the skeleton has no power of its own to maintain the figure in an upright position on the earth. The spirit, which has formed the skeleton in its own image, makes use of it as an instrument for walking and standing.

Human consciousness is also necessary for man to manifest himself. Just as the ego-organization needs the mineral skeleton as a foundation for standing and walking, so the ego-organization needs mineral substances in all the organs in order to develop the earthly consciousness. A child is feeble-minded when it is unable to form brain-sand (this is what the minerals enclosed in the pineal gland are called). Sodium, potassium and calcium are the necessary mineral constituents of the blood and the various organs for the right earthly consciousness.

The consciousness can only connect itself in the right way with the spirit when it has this mineral foundation in the body. This is where the other aspect of the 'U' is manifest: the longing for the spirit, the fervent aspiration towards the spirit. If a person is firmly anchored in the right way in his body, then he may go beyond himself to ardent spiritual experience. In 'U' there is a tremendous range of degrees of warmth, from the numbing coldness in which the dead bones can be formed, to the warmest spiritual inwardness, the utmost inward warmth of spirit. In a person who is ill we can very often see how both disintegrate. The lower limbs are not penetrated sufficiently, are heavy and tired. Varicose veins and dropsy develop. Dropped arches, prolapse of the organs of the lower body or the digestive tract occurs; the lower being falls a prey to weight. The activity does not penetrate into the body, nor does it give adequate support for the mind. Illusory ideas, whims and fancies hinder an objective union with the spirit. Subjection to the forces of gravity correspond to an ineffective life of the spirit.

In the 'U'-exercise the two sides must not fall apart. Care must be taken when doing 'U' for malformation of the figure, e.g. for knock-knees or bow-legs, that it is not only the stiffening power of 'U' that takes effect. The result is then achieved in the wrong way. Inwardness of spirit should be our guide when we undertake postural corrections. We must pay particular attention to a careful observation of the feet. The numerous malformations or formlessness of the feet is quite alarming. The heels are like lumps, the feet are not articulated and the various joints in the feet are inflexible, the toes are formless, the arch of the foot is not elastic. Even in old people there are cases where the feet no longer serve their purpose of standing properly—they get hard and horny. These are symptoms of the deterioration of the forces of elasticity. The legs and feet are no longer humanly permeated, as we have described it in the 'U'-gesture.

The significance of the feet for the whole organism and the seriousness of the situation as regards general health is clearly described in an article by Prof. Thomson (see Appendix, p. 174).

Also when powers of thought and memory are weak, for dizziness and eye troubles (short-sightedness, astigmatism), it is particularly important that the formative movement should work right down and into the feet. Here it is the diametrically opposite activity that is having the effect, which we know: exercises with the feet have a beneficial effect on the upper being and vice versa. It is just such polar opposite effects that we are using when we apply a metamorphosed 'U'-exercise against tics. Tics are involuntary, uncontrolled reflex movements which can be located anywhere, e.g. the eye-lid, the corner of the mouth or in the limbs. They are movements which come from the astral body without ego control. We have two exercises for this condition.

'U'—with the feet firmly on the ground, rising on to the toes and slowly lowering again, 12 times.

'U'—with the arms aiming at something, e.g. from high up down to shoulder level, or upwards to the tip of the nose—or else aiming at something in the room (running with 'U' to the window or the door etc.)—all as quick as lightning.

The slow raising and lowering of the feet puts a great strain on the legs; the ego is called upon to enter strongly into the limb movement. There is, too, an appeal to the ego in the aiming exercises—the involuntary movements can be overcome by strengthening the ego.

In practising with patients suffering from a tic, it can also be observed that there is a certain lack of strength in the feet. Sometimes the gait is halting, sometimes hasty, often the legs are stiff.

If 'U' is too difficult to begin with in these ailments, and the feet are cold and inflexible, then other exercises may be done first, e.g. 'A' is done for a longish period and is followed up later with 'U'.

Children who need 'U' can also be introduced to it by means of balancing copper rods, playing with copper balls; they can be encouraged to jump more, or when playing in the fields to pick flowers with their toes until the little foot is so supple and warm and relaxed that 'U' can give it the right form to harden into. To keep on practising again and again, to see whether one can stand for a long time on the heels or the toes, or whether one can do an 'I' with each toe—this is not a waste of time for grown-ups either.

The chilling, mineralizing tendency of 'U' can only work in the right way when a burning desire to get back to the original source is flowing through the gesture, thereby giving the body youthful elasticity and the soul courage to stand upright in life.

One says: 'an upright man'—this is taken to mean a person who remains loyal to his inner ideals and does not allow himself to be cast down by life's difficulties and hindrances.

The connection between the activity of the ego-organization in the material and in the spiritual heights is brought about by one organ within us, the spleen. It is formed by the system of forces belonging to Saturn. The sound 'U' comes from the same region. The spleen is regarded as an organ not essential to life, for it can be surgically removed without endangering life. Several little new ones are formed. This shows the vitality and strength of the regenerative forces of this organ. The spleen is included in the digestive tract, as are the liver and gall-bladder, though it is not so much concerned with the change of *substance* (*Stoff*wechsel) nor with the *change* of substance (Stoff*wechsel*), as with the regulation of certain rhythms. (*Stoffwechsel* is the German word for 'digestion'.) It changes the un-rhythm with which we take in food into a rhythm that is required by the blood circulation. Un-rhythm is changed into rhythm. For how would the organism endure if what is taken in so irregularly as food were to enter the blood-stream just as irregularly? We are sustained by the regular rhythm of the blood which has its precise relationship to the breathing. In *Occult Physiology* Rudolf Steiner has much to say about the spleen. We get some idea of how far we are from understanding an organ if we only know the physical part of it. This piece of 'cosmic astrality', which as the spleen lies so small and so unobtrusively in the upper left side of the abdomen, is an organ filled with spiritual light. It is a transformer of rhythms—cosmic rhythms are changed into earthly-organic rhythms. These rhythms, however, do not enter our consciousness; we do not recognize them yet. 'They differ quite considerably from other rhythms of which we are already aware.' The spleen serves to regulate 'what goes on inside the human being between the crude digestion and what is taking place in a more spiritual, ensouled way'. We may therefore regard the spleen as an organ that is lodged in the digestive tract as a sense organ, to enable the spiritual part of man to perceive the injurious effects of what is unrhythmical in the digestion. There is also another important function belonging to the spleen, namely, the active instinct as to the value of what we eat; that is to say, about the fitness of the quality of our food. This takes place deep down in the subconsciousness. Here we see highest spirituality concealed deep down within the organic activity. The spleen belongs—as already mentioned—to the forces working from Saturn. The formation of the physical body began on Old Saturn. The instincts are important for us as gifts from the gods—gifts which belong exclusively to the physical body. In the animal kingdom they work right down into the fitting construction of their habitations. The beaver does not have to learn how to make its lodge—it knows instinctively from out of its physical body. Through the development of consciousness man has lost the vitality of instinct. But deep within him, shut away from the consciousness, the instinct for the evaluation of substance works in the spleen. This organ is there like a warden, controlling the rhythms and evaluating the substances. At the present time especially, the instinct for the quality of food has been lost. Therefore the confusion about the different methods of nutrition gets worse and worse. The efforts to 'improve' natural foodstuffs with additives and preservatives would not have succeeded so well if a healthy instinct for the right food had been at work. How important it is, then, to stimulate the activity of the spleen, and to strengthen the instinct. Rudolf Steiner advises for this light massage of the spleen which, however, must be undertaken with great care, otherwise the opposite effect is induced. In this connection we could also think of doing regular practice of the 'U'-exercise which in this case would be deemed to be a hygienic-therapeutic measure. The first exercise that springs to mind is the 'U'-exercise which we know as one of the soul exercises: 'Hope-U'. To begin with we express in a gesture of eurythmy the feeling of desire, of hope. Through it we experience the lower organism as a vessel. The legs stand parallel, the feet planted firmly on the heels, while the toes gently leave the floor. The arms form a bowl-shape. This gesture goes over in a 'U'-movement. After a pause in the position of balance we start again with the hope-gesture and conclude it again with 'U'. 'This has a warming effect on the breathing system'—is what is said in the Curative Eurythmy Course. This phrase, difficult for modern medical thinking to accept, becomes comprehensible when we bear in mind the activity of the spleen in transforming the rhythms and of bringing the metabolic warmth in the right way into the blood circulation and the breathing.

This also makes the use of 'U' in cases of insomnia caused by digestive upsets understandable.

CHAPTER 5

Vowel Sequences

The composition and the physiological effect of the vowel sequences 'A-E-I-O-U' is discussed in various passages. The first two sounds, 'A' and 'E', help the soul and spirit to come into the physical body; they assist the process of incarnation. In mood they have a minor character in contrast to 'O' and 'U' which have a major character mood, and which help to raise the soul and spirit out of the organic system; they assist the process of excarnation. 'I' stands in the middle between these two.

'A-E-I-O-U' for stammering

With this vowel sequence it should be noted that one begins with 'A' and 'E', the incarnating sounds, and then lays particular stress on 'I' because it is the turning point leading to the excarnation sounds of 'O' and 'U'. It brings about stronger and more relaxed breathing. The vowel sequence is combined with hexameter rhythms.

The exercise can be done in the following way: we go backwards with 'A', 'E' and 'I', changing the caesura from the left accentuation of 'I' to the right, and then go forwards with 'I', 'O' and 'U'—all in hexameter rhythm. The changeover from 'U' to 'A' takes place when standing at the front. (See Chapter 6.)

Besides the harmonizing for the breath there are other exercises which we use for stammering and which we have to discover from the nature of the impediment. It depends especially on which consonants cannot be formed properly.

We have the exercise 'G-K-A-I' for a child who had trouble with the gutteral sounds.

Rudolf Steiner also suggested that sentences should be made up using the consonants which the child cannot say without stammering. The child says these sentences while walking, and the same consonants are also done in eurythmy. Rudolf Steiner added that nervous stammering in childhood often disappears later on and need not be taken too seriously.

For kleptomania

'All vowels with the legs'. This phrase comes from the Curative Education Course. In it Rudolf Steiner describes the nature of kleptomania as follows: '. . . then the intellectual capacity slips down into the will and kleptomania may ensue'. Through practising the vowels with the legs 'the intellectual element is driven out of the will and the striving, the effort, that lies in the vowel sounds, is impelled into the will'.

It is also good to jump the vowels rapidly with the legs. Poems suitable here are, above all, humorous ones.

Rudolf Steiner gave the following advice for a 12-year-old boy with kleptomania. 'We can now begin curative eurythmy with him. You should really have some strong garters made for him, to be bound tightly round his leg just below the knee. And then, when he is wearing these, he should do "A" with a jump, and indeed in such a way that both legs are bent at the knee, and also with his toes. So it is chiefly this leg exercise with "A". And then he should also do "E" with a jump. And for the present we could let him do it the whole day long.'

'Kleptomania-E'. Sitting with crossed legs, the arms are also crossed so that the toes can be grasped with the opposite hand. The child should remain for 10–15 minutes in this position.

Literally it is said: 'He should be made to sit there for a quarter of an hour holding on to his feet with his hands as a punishment.' This exercise should be continued for three months. And further:

'The memory is strengthened by backwards imagination, e.g.

> Father reads a book—
> Book a reads father,

also numbers back to front: 3426–6243, or the hardness-scale backwards and forwards. Speech exercises done backwards, too.'

For children who have a propensity for stealing it is always important to practise remembering back. It is suggested that 'thieving children should be made to remember what they have gone through in previous years. Let them imagine things from past years. Otherwise they can develop later on into kleptomaniacs'.

The following explanation by Rudolf Steiner shows that we must use the vowels to their fullest effect in order to strengthen the individuality of the child:

> Where there is kleptomania it is really like this: a human being has this polar opposite organization. It is the nature of the head organization to appropriate

everything to itself, it has to get everything for itself. The head organization is the one pole, while the other pole, the digestive organization, carries the moral sense. This can even be drawn diagramatically, with a lemniscate. The head organization does not know what ownership entails; it only knows about possessing everything coming within its reach. The other pole knows the moral aspect. Kleptomania arises when the organization of the head simply slips down into the will organization. What underlies this illness is that a person has in his will organization the elements which properly belong to the head organization. Quite different from these kleptomanic tendencies which are characterized by absence of mind during the act of stealing—it is more the material appearance of the object to be stolen which catches the eye, rather than the article itself which is the temptation, no artful ruses are practised to obtain the object . . . the image of kleptomania is very limited.

The words 'quite different' refer here to the contrast between kleptomanic stealing and ordinary stealing.

For epilepsy

'A' and 'E'. These two vowels which are the main exercise for epilepsy have already been discussed in Chapter 4.

'All vowels with the legs'. These were prescribed for a 43-year old epileptic patient who had suffered from fits since his 29th year. In these attacks the convulsions chiefly affected the upper part of the body and the face, and Rudolf Steiner said: 'We are dealing here with a very weak astral body. The etheric body goes into the upper part and out to the periphery, and then a kind of inner worry comes up that the etheric body may escape altogether, and therefore, the condition arises.'

'Vowels with feet and legs'. These were prescribed for a 46-year-old epileptic patient.

'Using the vowels'

'I' (as complete curative eurythmy exercise)—
'E' (as complete curative eurythmy exercise)—

These were all done with an 18-year-old epileptic patient who had had convulsive movements of the hand since his seventh year, and at the age of 11 had had his first epileptic fit. The patient found the curative eurythmy so helpful that he returned after an interval when he did not feel very well. Each time the whole 'E'-exercise was performed, then the vowels and then the whole 'I'-exercise.

Otosclerosis

'Vowels with the legs'. In otosclerosis we are dealing with the formation of spongy bone in the capsule of the labyrinth. The porous, blood-filled bone becomes hardened and it can also lead to hardening of the oval window of the vestibule, whereby the stapes becomes fixed. Moreover, a degenerative process of the hearing and of the equilibrium nerve makes its appearance. The illness usually commences between 20 and 30 years of age and appears more frequently in women than in men. It is often worse during pregnancy.

These hardening forces, working too strongly in the head, are loosened when activity and consciousness are brought into the limbs through the vowels. It will often be noticed that these patients quickly get the hang of an exercise; they execute the movements with the legs with skill and aptitude, and can run rhythms easily, but it is all 'thought out' excessively. For this reason one likes to do poems with changing rhythms and not stay too long with one poem.

Nowadays this illness can be treated by surgery. But it should be clearly understood that the constitution is not thereby altered at all and patients still need to do this exercise.

'General use of vowels'

This has been suggested in the Curative Eurythmy Course for many disorders, some of which have already been mentioned with the particular vowels. The vowels are used especially for *irregular breathing*, because with them we work particularly strongly upon the rhythmic system.

'General use of vowels'. For children who have *difficulty in speaking certain consonants*—especially labial sounds and dental sounds. We can help to overcome the difficulties with the quiet use of vowels.

'General use of vowels'. For children and adults who suffer from *chronic headaches, migraine conditions*, and for those who complain of *giddiness* or *drowsiness*, or who tend to have a *sluggish digestion*.

'Vowel curative eurythmy' was prescribed by Rudolf Steiner for a 45-year-old man who had had a *nervous breakdown*, and in consequence suffered from insomnia and could no longer control his thoughts. At times 'the head thought by itself, that is, it was automatic'. At a later stage, trembling limbs and convulsive conditions appeared. After taking an equisetum bath he had to do vowels in curative eurythmy *for a whole hour*. What was started by the bath 'is impelled, through curative eurythmy towards the tendency to become permanent'. It can be seen that curative eurythmy is given here in a large dose and is allowed to tire the patient. [21 January 1924.]

'General use of vowels' was also prescribed for the onset of *schizophrenia*. This is understandable since the vowels strengthen the human being in himself and bring harmony between the various members of his being. They bring him to himself as a human being.

'General use of vowels' for children who *'are tormented by their imagination'*. Rudolf Steiner gave this exercise for children with too much imagination with whom it works particularly well if, besides using the vowels, the whole body is brought into movement through running, stepping and walking. In this way the images, stirred up out of the organism, are mollified. On the other hand, children who have too little imagination should do the consonants in eurythmy while standing still. [15 June 1921.]

The following is a specialized exercise:

Monday: only the sound 'I' in eurythmy
Tuesday: only the sound 'E'
Wednesday: only the sound 'O'
Thursday: only the sound 'U'
Friday: only the sound 'A'
Saturday: the whole word—without ever speaking it aloud

Each time it was practised for 10-15 minutes.

Frau L. Meyer-Smits was given this exercise in 1916, before there was any curative eurythmy in existence, for a dreamy child of about 9 years old, who was backward at school and 'not quite with it'. Frau Meyer-Smits kindly gave permission for it to be published.

'I-A-O'

Of the vowel exercises which do not include the whole sequence, the most important is 'I-A-O'.

One after the other the upper part of the body is stretched up in 'I', 'A' is jumped with the legs, and 'O' is formed with the arms on a level with the heart, and all three sounds are held together at the same time. Then first the 'O' is let go, then 'A' and finally 'I'—and begin again from the beginning. Gradually the exercise is accelerated until all three sounds are formed simultaneously, then the tempo is slowed down again.

'I-A-O' brings harmony to the threefold human being—to the head system, to the digestive-limb system and to the rhythmic system—and can be regarded as a transition leading over to hygienic eurythmy.

The consonance of the sounds 'I-A-O' is very important; in olden times it sounded forth as 'I-O-A' to the pupils of the Mystery Schools, in order to direct their gaze towards what lay before birth. In the Mysteries of Ephesus one experienced in the initiation ceremony into the Mystery of the goddess Diana how 'I' sounded forth as the individuality descended, 'O' as the spirit clothed itself with the soul, and 'A' as the etheric body was drawn in. Today we no longer have 'I-O-A' but instead we have 'I-A-O'—this is appropriate for our time. The descent of mankind from the spiritual into the physical world has been accomplished. The soul and spirit of man have completely permeated the body, and now the danger threatens that they become too firmly embedded in the body. So now the problem is to free the soul again and to connect it with its surroundings; from its lowest point to set it again on the upward path to the spiritual world. We do this when we experience ourselves spiritually ('I') in our body ('A') and with 'O' we again make visible the distinctive characteristics of the soul. What in earlier times was known only in the secret Mysteries through the sounding forth of 'I-O-A' today has become a common exercise which may be performed by anyone. However, Rudolf Steiner points out that it should not be done by the class as a whole in the schools, but that it is better to form a group of those children out of the various classes in whom it is obvious that the three parts of the human being are not in harmony with one another. It is important that this significant exercise should always be newly worked out as a hygienic-therapeutic exercise. Further details of the various possibilities of how to form the 'I-A-O' exercise are to be found in *Eurythmy Therapy in Practice* by E. Baumann.

'T-I-A-O-A-I-T'

This exercise which is built up as a palindrome brings order to disordered, 'muddled' thinking and has therefore general hygienic usefulness.

'A-O-U-M'

The ancient Indian syllable 'AOUM' was given in earlier times by the recognized leaders of mankind to those who were younger as an effective exercise to 'train them to be physically whole men and at the same time to be discreet'. This vowel sequence, which is significantly concluded with 'M', affects the regulation of the breathing with the emphasis on exhalation.

'L-A-O-U-M'

This has proved in practice to be beneficial in cases of *asthma* and *glaucoma*. In both these conditions outbreathing has to be stimulated. To begin with 'L' intensifies the drawing-in of the breath and thereby strengthens the effect on the outbreathing.

'A-E-I—I-E-A'

For children who *lack powers of imitation*. The power to imitate is a great gift which man brings with him from the spiritual world where he turned towards the higher beings in devoted imitation. The lack of this faculty occasions great difficulties for the whole development of a child. We find these failings sometimes in retarded children who have trouble with walking, speaking and thinking—the three human faculties which are developed during the first period of life. These children show no inclination to enter properly into the physical body, 'they can scarcely overcome the desire of their physical body for peace and quiet'. These children should do tone eurythmy first, in order to stimulate some sort of inner movement; then eurythmy and speech exercises, slowly forwards and backwards. 'A-E-I—I-E-A' belongs to these exercises. The power of imitation diminishes at the approach of the ninth year; if this does not take place satisfactorily and the child retains too much of the imitative power, then 'I'-exercises may be used to strengthen the ego. [Curative Education Course.]

'E-U-Ö'

This is for a bodily and mentally *retarded* child.
 For this condition also speech exercises forwards and backwards are done, in order to regulate the relationship between the etheric and astral bodies and 'exercises in curative eurythmy which help the child to experience his own physical organization. 'E' is particularly suitable for this, since here a human being touches himself in his organization; the same applies to 'U' and 'Ö'. 'Ö' is used as a regulator. There was a child of almost 7 years who had a very irregular digestion, a voracious appetite

'I', 'U', 'E'

To arouse the *sensibility of the body* in a girl in the Waldorf School in Stuttgart. She did not want to listen to any fairy-stories or poems, and showed amoral inclinations.

The instructions were: 'I' with the whole body, 'U' with the index finger on the ears, 'E' with the hair, and all three sounds so that they 'contain some sensibility'.

'U', 'O', 'I'

For Little's disease. A 15-year-old girl who had a mild form of this disease had splay feet on both sides. She learnt to walk when she was 3 years old. She could, however, only walk on tiptoe and could not keep her balance. There was no improvement in her walking even after an operation to sever the Achilles tendon. For her Rudolf Steiner laid the greatest importance on curative eurythmy. He recommended threefold walking forwards, and also especially backwards, with arms at an angle, the upper arm pressed tightly to the body, the fists clenched—followed by the whole 'U'-exercise, the whole 'O'-exercise and the whole 'I'-exercise. This last exercise was to be done in such a way that she stood on one leg only, alternatively left and right. In addition she was to describe a circle with the right foot while standing on the left leg, and the same with the left foot while standing on the right leg.

'I-E-Ei'

Rudolf Steiner gave this exercise for a child who was in danger of becoming ill with *tuberculosis of the pancreas*. Unfortunately the child had the treatment for only a very short time, so we are unable to say anything about the effect of this exercise.

CHAPTER 6

Basic Exercises in Curative Eurythmy

Various factors will now be discussed which are not, strictly speaking, part of curative eurythmy, but which, nevertheless, can be considered as supplementary to the curative eurythmy exercises, strengthening them and supporting them.

Some of the exercises that will be described can also be used where curative eurythmy as such would not be appropriate, for instance, in so-called hygienic eurythmy, or in factories where eurythmy is done to mitigate the harmful effects of industrial life. Frau Dr Wegman took a particular interest in this hygienic eurythmy. She said many times in conversation that the bodies of the civilized peoples were getting harder and were, therefore, hostile to the spirit. And so she wished that hygienic eurythmy should be developed so that the body could, once again, become permeated by the spirit. This appeared to her to be particularly important for the countries of Western Europe and America.

To counteract the ill-effects of industry it is enough—according to Rudolf Steiner—to do 15 minutes eurythmy daily. In factories it should be done all together as a community, as indeed is already the case in some anthroposophical undertakings.

If we want to go into detail now, we must head the list with the basic exercise of slow, threefold walking. It comes up in every curative eurythmy lesson if the patient is able to walk at all. To everyone actively engaged in curative eurythmy, the way a patient walks is an important diagnostic clue, and in eurythmic walking we have an intensified expression of the human being.

The first phase of this kind of walking—loosening the foot from the ground—is a will-movement in which the higher members of the being penetrate into the physical body and etheric body and, in overcoming weight, raise the foot. The second phase is carrying the foot; this is a raising up out of the forces of gravity with which the thought, preceding the resolve to walk, can unite itself. In the third phase, placing the foot, we touch down upon the ground again in a loving deed. In so doing the higher members are released once more, so that they may penetrate again in the next lifting of the foot. The harmonious performance of these three phases, lifting, carrying and placing the foot, is in itself a completely healing exercise. At the same time to experience in the centre of the breast the point of balance which keeps us poised, enabling us to carry the head freely and to move forwards and backwards smoothly and surely, are accomplishments not always easy to perform.

But the illness often becomes visible when doing this threefold walking. For instance, a depressive person will be very reluctant and tentative in the first phase of lifting his foot from the ground—a person who is afraid will try to cut as short as possible the free swing of the second phase—and the indifferent, unconscious placing of the foot reveals how difficult it is for that person to connect himself with the earth in a truly human way. Haste in the third phase can, in an illness such as paralysis, which is connected with absent-mindedness, lead to complete instability where random movements in all directions make it impossible for the foot to touch the ground purposefully. These are only a few examples to stimulate closer and better observation of the quite individual process of walking in every human being.

It could, however, be therapeutically desirable to emphasize particularly one of these three phases—whether it be the lifting, carrying or placing of the foot—but it would always be a good idea to finish with the harmonious triad of threefold walking as such.

From walking forwards and backwards we come to the ego-line through which we strengthen the power of the ego, for in the ego there lies 'the pointing back to oneself—the concept of the self-turned-inwards-towards-the-self'. The essential point about the ego-line is that in walking backwards one must step again exactly in the footsteps made in going forwards.

A variation of the ego-line is to do the exercise beginning with two steps forwards and backwards, then three steps, four, five, six up to seven, and then down again, six, five, four, three, two steps. And at the same time the tempo is changed according to the rule 'slow, becoming fast—fast, becoming slow'.

The following simple exercise can be developed out of walking: three steps forward are taken at an even pace, but the third step is replaced with a jerking check of the upper body. In the next three steps the middle step is left out in the same way, and in the following three steps the first step is left out—then from the beginning again. This exercise brings about a taking-hold-of-oneself; the astrality is curbed by the ego. Many variations can be found of the same principles.

So far we have only considered going forwards and backwards, but now we come to the running of forms. The following is a simple but very effective exercise: walking backwards energetically with the thought 'I will'; then, with relaxed legs and feet, walking forwards on the same line with 'I cannot'; then walking in a circle with 'I must', whereby in the rounded form the will forces are engaged in the right way.

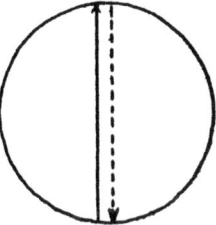

In this exercise the circle can be felt as something harmoniously making up for the one-sidedness of the previous forms and linking us with the powers of the circumference.

In order to bring the experience of movement as such to sick people, it is often necessary to let them run forms. A good exercise here is the simple polarity of 'the outer has triumphed' and 'the inner has triumphed'.

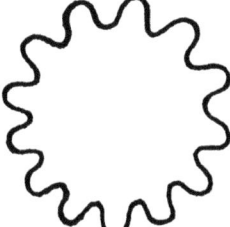　　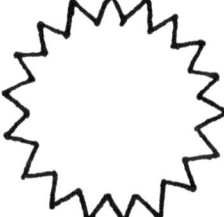

'The inner has triumphed'　　'The outer has triumphed'

It is necessary to comprehend space in terms of all geometrical forms, such as triangle, pentagram, six-pointed star, circle, etc. to bring consciousness into the limbs, to create clarity and harmony in a human being.

The pentagram, which restores the etheric form of the human being, is often combined with the five vowel sounds, or with 'Hallelujah', which is used in curative eurythmy to strengthen and sustain the etheric—this can readily be appreciated from the meaning of the word 'Hallelujah': 'I purify myself of all that prevents me from beholding the Divine.'

The lemniscate form, often in conjunction with the harmonizing 'L-M', or the harmonious eight, are used where the sense of movement and skill in movement have to be stimulated, as for instance, is the case with cancer patients.

If various forms are directly linked together with each other, this strengthens the etheric body and makes it resilient. To give an example: ego-line, run as the centre axis of a lemniscate. The various forms can be accompanied by contrasting rhythms which intensifies the effect. For instance, a pentagram is run to an anapaest and it is enclosed within a circle to dactyl.

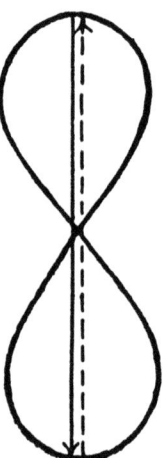

The whole wealth of Dionysian and Apollonian forms may be drawn upon when it is a question of putting vowels or consonants to spatial forms. Usually, of course, this does not mean making use of the whole new choreography of artistic forms which Rudolf Steiner created for artistic eurythmy. But the basic principles underlying the Dionysian forms, for instance, can be recognized: that the soul-forces of thinking, feeling and willing can be separated according to their inherent difference, and each experienced for itself in its own sphere—this can enliven and quicken people whose souls have become stiff and numb, or those whose thinking, feeling and willing are too closely knit together or liable to disintegrate.

The Apollonian forms, with their precise grammatical construction, may be used for people who are too introspective, as in neurasthenia, or also for people who have tendencies towards diseases of deposition. By means of these forms they can experience grammatical regularity being transformed into movement.

The inward and outward winding spirals also belong to the forms which may be run as curative eurythmy exercises. The inward spiral is given for anaemic children to strengthen their ego organically, and to stimulate the formation of blood—also to strengthen consciousness of self. With the arms, either the gesture '*Schau in Dich*' (Look into thyself) may be done with it, or a movement starting with 'A' and going over into an 'E'. The outward spiral, on the other hand, is performed with full-blooded children who are too egocentric and might be prone to outbursts of temper. In this case the form is accompanied by the arm movement for '*Schau um Dich*' (Look around thee), or else, starting with the gesture for 'E', it is led over into an 'A' or even a 'U'.

As an exercise for the soul in entering into and withdrawing from the body, the inward spiral leads directly into the outward spiral, or the form for '*Schau in Dich—Schau um Dich*' is run.

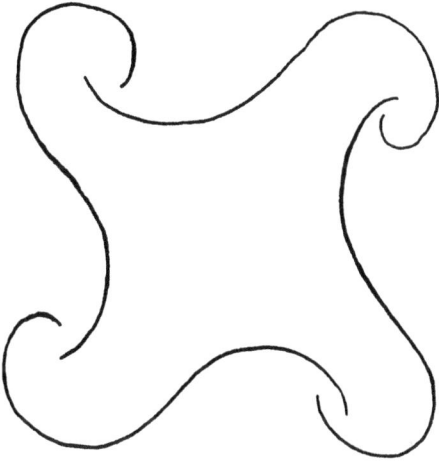

We will now say something briefly about postures of the body. To begin with we have the meditation exercise for eurythmy, '*Ich denke die Rede*', by means of which one prepares oneself for eurythmy and which is, therefore, often done at the beginning or at the end of the eurythmy lesson. We cannot do justice to its full significance here, but nevertheless we will refer to Rudolf Steiner's words: 'These gestures, when carried out in this way one after the other, form an exercise which may be classed among those having a harmonizing and curative effect upon the soul. That is to say, when anyone is so deeply disturbed in his soul-life that this is also outwardly perceptible in the body, manifesting itself in various digestive disorders, then, as a curative eurythmy exercise this is the one above all others which may be given with the greatest benefit.' This is an exercise which can also often be applied with success for ailments which occur at the climacteric to facilitate the change in position of the warmth pole which takes place at this time.

In a lecture on the Rosicrucians, Rudolf Steiner gave the exercise '*Licht strömt aufwärts—Schwere lastet abwärts*' (Light streams upwards—Weight bears downwards). The upper triangle is formed

Light streams upwards

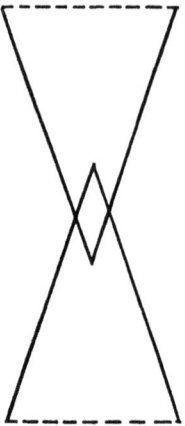

Weight bears downwards

with the arms and the horizontal connection has to be felt from hand to hand—and the same with the lower triangle which is formed with the legs and the connection felt from foot to foot. When the forces of lightness in the soul are too firmly embedded in the organism, the exercise can be used to loosen them. In doing the exercise there is a tremendous awakening of consciousness in the region of the solar plexus where the two triangles overlap. Therefore this exercise is also important for strengthening and soothing this centre of the vegetative nervous system.

Now besides these aspects which concern the whole body, we also have those which are performed by the head only, or by the feet only. The head positions which Rudolf Steiner gave for artistic eurythmy can also be used now and again in curative eurythmy. Since we know that movements of the head frequently have their effect in the lower being, for example, in the curative eurythmy exercise which we know as 'M with head-shaking', we can use the same when it is a question of influencing the lower being. So that 'E' made with the eyes—that is, squinting inwards—is given as an exercise to restore harmony in the abdomen.

Conversely, foot positions can be used to work upon the upper being. There are two foot exercises which are well known as curative eurythmy exercises: 'Yes and No' and 'Sympathy and Antipathy', both of which are fully described in the Curative Eurythmy Course.

We come now to the question of rhythm. The action of rhythm takes place in the alternation of long and short beats—this can be carried out in eurythmy either by beating time with the arms or with the legs in running. Even if the patient is only able to do it with the hands—by making a slight, indistinct curve, and on the long beat stretching out the fingers in a more clearly defined movement—this has an effect on the blood-breath rhythm in the region of the breast of the person. The actual healer in the human being is situated in this region where blood and breath meet. There a person really is human. From Rudolf Steiner we know that original human speech was not arrhythmical prose, but of necessity came forth in a rhythmical flow. Human life was created out of cosmic life-rhythms, and hidden within it the mystery of rhythm lives on in a multitude of ways—in the pulse beat, in the breathing, in the rhythmic processes of digestion, in the ebb and flow of the cerebral fluid.

In the course of the earth's evolution man has left further and further behind him this state of being embedded in the cosmic-rhythmical processes so that he could bring the ego to birth in freedom. In this way rhythm today is frequently overpowered by the chaos of arrhythm, and indeed, even of anti-rhythm.

> But it is also essential that man should not think that he can live without rhythm. As he has become an inward being from without, so he must build himself up again rhythmically from within. That is the important thing. Rhythm must permeate the inner being. Just as rhythm has built up the cosmos, so man must become permeated with a new rhythm if he is to take part in building up a new cosmos. It is characteristic of the times in which we live that the old rhythm—the outer one—has been lost and no new, inner rhythm has yet been found. Man has grown away from Nature—if we call the outward expression of the Spirit, Nature—and has not yet grown into the Spirit itself. At the moment he is left suspended between Nature and Spirit. That is what is characteristic of our times. And this floundering to and fro between Nature and Spirit reached its climax in the second third of the nineteenth century. And therefore, round about that time, the beings who know and interpret the signs of the times had to put the question: What is to be done in order that mankind shall not fall out of rhythm altogether, that an inner rhythm may enter into him?

Rudolf Steiner spoke thus earnestly in a lecture 'Rhythms in Man's Nature'. [12 January 1909.]

From these words it will be obvious how much depends upon mankind learning to live in inner rhythm. Of course, that goes far beyond the study of rhythms as we use them in the field of curative eurythmy—but it is still good to carry the idea within oneself as a thought, of the widest and all-embracing rhythm, out of which man is to create a new cosmos in order to kindle from this ideal concept within oneself, as a curative eurythmist, the enthusiasm to induce people to immerse themselves in the right way in the healing element of rhythm.

If we now consider the essential nature of rhythm, we find it, as we have already said, in the alternation of long and short beats. In Grecian culture—the original birthplace of harmonious human existence and thus of rhythm as well—there used to be a rhythm consisting of long beats only. If one can submerge oneself in this rhythm, as a kind of exercise, then one can experience how the outbreathing is activated from the head, but it could also lead to stupor. There was also a rhythm consisting of short beats only. In the echo of this rhythm one feels caught up and exhausted in a struggle that never comes to a restful conclusion, but gets held up in inhalation. Both rhythms are instructive in their one-sidedness, but they are untherapeutic and are therefore only seldom used in curative eurythmy. Healing is to be found in the alternation of long and short beats.

So on the one hand we have all the variations of rhythm which begin with a short beat and flow into the long beat—the iambic measure. With it the will can be fired and the rhythm of the blood is made to beat more rapidly. From the iambic group of rhythms one can be chosen for sluggishness of the circulation and also of the digestion, but it should be remembered that iambic rhythms, as such, affect the will system more than anapaestic rhythms which work in a more delicate, stimulating way upon the inner soul-life.

The group of trochiac measures, which begin with a long beat, work soothingly and deepen exhalation. People from the big cities who are always hurrying and rushing about will need these trochaic rhythms—whereby it should be noted that the trochaic, as such, works from the head, calming the thoughts, while the dactylic rhythm, on the other hand, works more into the innermost soul and brings calm breathing to nervous agitation. It should, however, be noted that it is often necessary to tackle what is working one-sidedly in a person with the same, before it can be transformed into the opposite. Thus, it might be necessary to let a person who is nervous and restless start with iambic rhythms before going on to trochee which, in certain circumstances, might be so foreign to his nature that at first he would not be able to tolerate it.

Rudolf Steiner has succeeded in putting into effect the healer's principle 'like works upon like' in the two rhythms which he gave for curative eurythmy: curative eurythmy iambus and trochee.

The curative eurythmy iambus always starts on the left with a big step—then the right follows with a long step which is made in a quiet, positive manner, then comes a pause in which the arms are brought to rest. Thus there are three underlying units here: (i) a long, energetic step from the left and an arm movement representing half an 'A', (ii) the long beat and completion of the 'A' with the right arm, (iii) rest position. Having regard to the disorder to be treated, namely fidgetiness, this metamorphosis of iambus is easily understood. A fidgety child energetically starts doing all sorts of things only to leave them again immediately and turn his attention to something else. In the exercise his energy is met by the first energetic step—then follows (infinitely salutory) the completion from the right, soothing and positive, then restraint in the pause. It does a restless child good to help him unobtrusively to finish something which he has begun. This attitude also underlies our curative eurythmy exercise.

For the phlegmatic child the curative eurythmy trochee is used. This time we start with the right, again slowly forming half an 'A' with the right arm, and then the short left of the second phase follows as an awakening, stimulating movement. In this exercise any vowels may be used which seem to be necessary for the child. These two exercises are really curative, adapted to the illness. It should be noted here that the antispastic exercise with its 'short–long, long–short' beat can assist in reinforcing the cramp-releasing 'E'-exercise, since it works in a spasm-loosening way, as its name implies.

The following suggestions made by Rudolf Steiner can also be helpful in working with phlegmatic and sanguine children.

'Phlegmatic children can only be induced to move if an attempt is made to do the difficult consonants with them—with sanguine children, the easier ones. With the phlegmatics, "R" and "S". For the sanguine children, those consonants which start movement going: "D" and "T".'

We will now direct our attention to the hexameter measure, the rhythm that is founded on the same ratio of 4:1 as the pulse–breathing rhythm. Here the specific quality lies in the caesura: -vv-vv-vv/-vv-vv-vv. We use this rhythm for stammering. In stammering, the breathing is cramped, the transition from breathing-in to breathing-out is not effectual—that important moment in which the ego is intensely concerned. When the hexameter rhythm is performed in curative eurythmy, we usually do it together with the vowel sequence 'A-E-I-O-U'. What underlies this exercise is the connection of 'A' and 'E' with the minor experience of turning inwards upon oneself, and of 'O' and 'U' as a major experience of the desire to relate oneself to the outer world; and in between the 'I' as the turning point between being within and without (see also Chapter 5). The same procedure of going backwards in the minor mood can also be carried out with the tone eurythmy gestures for minor and major. This exercise is specially beneficial for respiratory disturbances in general, and can always be employed if the patient is able to use his legs for walking. The rhythmical 'R' is also often important in assisting relaxation, and of course, all rhythmical music in general.

*

And finally a word about rod exercises. In general it may be said that they discipline the body, and should make it pliant so that it can carry out

The sevenfold rod exercise

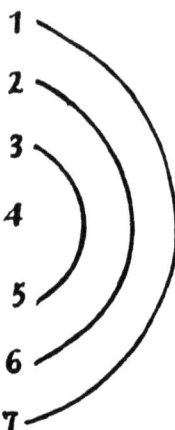

what is expected of it. Rod exercises are to correct faults in body posture, said Rudolf Steiner. These exercises verge on gymnastics—although they are not gymnastic exercises in the sense of toughening the body. It will be best if we turn to the individual exercises themselves in order to explain what is meant.

We have then the sevenfold rod exercise. From the way the diagram is drawn here, its mirror-picture construction may be recognized. The 'left' is roughly the middle of the exercise—'down, up, right, left' is like a tide swelling to the climax at 'left'—and then ebbing away again at 'right, up, down'. A musical crescendo and decrescendo is expressed in it. In order to become familiar with the qualities of the different directions in space, which is what underlies this exercise, reference should be made to Rudolf Steiner's explanations in *The Wisdom of Man, of the Soul and of the Spirit*.* Here we will just extract the scheme from this lecture:

> The streams of the physical body go from left to right—
> The streams of the ether body go from right to left—
> The streams of the sentient body go from front to back—
> The streams of the sentient soul go from back to front—
> The streams of the ego go from above downwards—
> The streams of the astral body go from below upwards—

The exercise begins with 'down' (this movement should be stressed, not just begun from 'down')—in this it addresses itself first to the ego which streams down in the vertical, and in this way, through the will, resists the force of gravity and overcomes it. 'Only when *will*, something

---

* Anthroposophic Press, New York 1971

spiritual, flows through the blood can the horizontal line turn into the vertical, can the upright carriage be attained and the group-soul be raised to the individual soul'—this is said in the same lecture as mentioned above. From 'down' it now goes 'up', that is, from the ego direction up into the direction of the astral body. Then follows 'right'. The streams of the physical body move towards the right. On the right side of the body we have the liver, our largest and most compact organ, which plays a big part in the transformation of thought into will. In the rod exercise the way from above towards the right should be strongly felt. Now follows the movement to the left. From right to left streams the etheric body, which lives in the forces of buoyancy, in lightness, and so we have the lighter organs also on the left-hand side of the body, such as the stomach and spleen. As this sevenfold rod exercise has a particular reference to the various directions of space it affects the physical body of man.

The twelvefold rod exercise is built up on strong rhythms and is, therefore, connected more with the etheric body. The pulse-breathing rhythm of 4:1 is concealed within it. When counting up to 12, the stressed accents come on 1, 4, 7, 10—that is, four accentuations to the 12 parts of the exercise.

The spiral is the prototype of astral movement and consequently this exercise works particularly upon the astral body. The blossom of the plant, which is influenced by cosmic astrality, opens and closes, often visibly, in spiral form; climbing plants twine themselves spirally round their support; the human astral body leaves the etheric body and physical body in spiral form on going to sleep and re-entering on waking up. These are only a few examples showing the connection of the astral with spiral movement.

Of all the rod exercises the 'Waterfall' is really *the* ego exercise—for the resolve to let go of the rod bravely has to be taken by the ego.

One can deduce from these indications when to use the one or the other exercise.

For enlivening and gaining control of the fingers and hand, the exercises '*Qui-qui*' and '*So-ist-es*' are mentioned, but it is not necessary to go into them further.

There are many other rod exercises which are adapable and useful in training the body in skill and accuracy. Rod practice stimulates the impulse to invent further exercises, and therefore there is a great abundance of them. One need only recall the numerous rod exercises for eye disorders or for special abnormalities of posture. However, only the main ones, given by Rudolf Steiner himself, have been discussed here.

CHAPTER 7

The Cosmic Aspect of the Vowels

The full significance of curative eurythmy can only be understood against the background of the anthroposophical knowledge of man. This does not look at man in isolation, but in relationship to the cosmos and to the kingdoms of Nature. Thus the phrase which used to ring out from the ancient wisdom of the Mysteries is again true: Man is the microcosm in the macrocosm and the macrocosm in the microcosm. In the old Mysteries, even until the Eleusinian and Ephesian Mysteries, one looked up to the cosmic Man who was created out of the primeval Word and in whom all creation was contained. Stars and the starry spheres were his organs, and the kingdoms of Nature were created with him. Even we ourselves are surrounded by the tradition of a connection with the whole universe. In old writings from the Middle Ages, and even as late as the nineteenth century, we find accounts of the congruity of the stars with formations in the realms of Nature and the various organs in man. It is from the seven main planets that everything derives: Sun, Moon, Mercury, Venus, Mars, Jupiter, Saturn. These planets are seen as having a connection with the origin of the chief metals, gold, silver, quicksilver, copper, iron, tin, lead; with plant groups; and with the seven main organs in man, heart, reproductive organs, lungs, kidneys, gall-bladder, liver and spleen. Even the days of the week show in their names their derivation from the planets: Sunday = Sun; Monday = Moon; Tuesday (French, Mardi, Italian, Martedi) = Mars; Wednesday (French, Mercredi, Italian, Mercoledi) = Mercury; Thursday, from Thor, the god of thunder, (Italian Giovedi) = Jupiter; Friday, from Teutonic, Frija, Frig (Italian, Venerdi) = Venus; Saturday = Saturn.

When we read the manuscripts that have come down to us, they may give us many an interesting indication, but they do not, in reality, alter our connection with the world around us. We do not thereby experience how our organs are formed out of the stars and how they, in their turn, work through the organs upon our life-processes and upon our various conditions of consciousness. Thus the traditional knowledge of the powers of the stars remains without meaning for us in our daily life.

Rudolf Steiner investigated cosmic man in a new way. He gives us a real picture of the various stellar spheres, of the deeds of spiritual beings and also of the experiences of human beings in these spheres. Human life then expands beyond the confines of birth and death. In the life after death the soul-spirit being passes from one stellar sphere to another, transforming the experiences of the previous earthly life—and returns by the same path before birth, preparing the next life on earth from what is experienced before birth. On his journey through the spheres, man builds up his inner organs according to the fruits of his previous life. 'If you were simply to make a diagram of a human being with his various organs, then his inner configuration—not, of course, the physical material which comes only at conception and birth—but his form, his inner organization, is the result of what he has lived through between death and a new birth ... Your heart, lungs, liver, are the products of what you experience between death and a new birth.' [*Anthroposophie als Kosmosophie.*]

The events which take place before birth in the various spheres and bring about the formation of our inner organs are described realistically and in great detail. For instance, during the time which the human being spends in the Sun-sphere he is working on the spirit-germ of his physical heart.

> Here he begins to separate himself off again as an individuality. Very faintly the feeling dawns that he is becoming separate from the Cosmos. This is connected with the fact that the first foundations of the heart are now being laid within him. The return journey continues. For the second time man passes through the Venus sphere and the Mercury sphere, where the spirit-germs of the other organs have to be implanted within him. At the moment of entrance for the second time into the Sun existence—at the moment when, out yonder in the Cosmos the spirit-germ of the heart is laid within our being on the return journey to the earth, there is, of course, not yet a physical heart. True, there is already an indication of a physical heart form, but it is surrounded and interwoven with all that constitutes the *worth* of the human being as the outcome of his previous earthly lives ... Before the spirit-germ of the heart unites with the embryonic germ of the future body, the heart in man is a spiritual being, a moral being of soul-and-spirit out in the Cosmos; only later does this moral being ... unite with the embryo. [*Supersensible Man.*]

Just as in the Sun-existence the spirit-germ of the heart is formed, so in each planetary sphere the germ of one of our inner organs comes into being:

in Saturn—the spleen
in Jupiter—the liver
in Mars—the gall-bladder
in the Sun—the heart

in Venus—the kidneys
in Mercury—the lungs
in the Moon—the brain and reproductive organs

The metals are to be regarded as substances which have solidified out of the activity of the planetary spheres, as cited at the beginning of the chapter. The vowels, as creative forces of the Word, are arranged in the following way as belonging to the planetary spheres: Sun = 'au', Venus = 'a', Mercury = 'i', Moon = 'ei', Mars = 'e', Jupiter = 'o', Saturn = 'u'.

All the organs—lungs, kidneys, spleen, etc.—have very different structures; the cells are specific and remain so throughout life although they are all nourished by the same blood. The organ can lose its appointed structure only in cases of illness, or infestation by foreign tissues. A hidden plan of construction must underlie each organ enabling it to ensure that its specific form is maintained. This is the archetypal image which has its origin in the planetary spheres.

*

We will take the kidneys and the spleen as an example and see if we can recognize in the gesture of the vowels the finer formative processes in the organ.

As paired organs the kidneys lie on either side of the spinal column. Seen in cross-section one is struck by the diffusion of the tubules and blood-vessels raying out from the kidney pelvis. From the bladder the ureters ascend at an angle to the kidneys. They are formed, even in the embryonic period, out of the cloaca and ascend from below to meet what comes down to them as rudiment of kidney and to combine with it. From the pelvis of the kidney they radiate in a number of angles to the periphery of the kidney. The microscopic picture of the kidney shows a clear division between the medullary substance and the cortex. In the medullary substance we recognize the gesture for 'A' in its ray-like structure. Coming from outside to meet the raying-out principle is an enveloping, stemming force which is seen in the cortex in the convolutions of blood vessels—called glomeruli—and in the twists of the uriniferous tubules. These blood gomeruli are enclosed by the Bowman's capsule. In the excretory, uriniferous tubules we find the raying-out principle in the ascending and descending straight tubules, while the stemming principle is in the convoluted tubules. The radiating power of 'A', which works through from the entrance to the kidney cortex, is clearly met by the enveloping gesture of 'B'. The microscope picture of the kidney gives, through the convolutions of the capillaries, an impression of something living and flourishing—comparable with a flowering rose hedge.

This is especially impressive when compared with the spleen. The spleen is like a sponge with its trabeculae of strong connective tissue and close network of elastic fibres. A firm capsule encloses the soft organ and between the layers of connective tissue lies the soft blood-mass of the splenic pulp from which the spongy tissue is formed. The peculiar thing about the blood vessels in the spleen is that they do not branch out at their extremities but run parallel to each other. The long, terminal ends lie stretched out together in bundles and are called arterioles. Just before they spread out they are united once more by a relatively thick outer covering and are then called sheathed arteries. They open into large cavities, the so-called splenic sinuses, where the closed-circuit of the blood ends. The blood dies here; only in the embryonic stage and in certain illnesses are red blood corpuscles formed here too. What a contrast to the picture of the kidneys! There we have a flowering process, while here we are looking at a process of death. The splenic sinuses, where aging blood gathers and is destroyed, are what give this impression. In the arterioles, with their remarkable contraction in the sheaths, we can easily recognize the gesture for 'U' in the power of contraction and in the parallelism.

*

In the etheric-physical part of the organs we see gesture which has frozen and come to an end. Also in the lungs, liver, gall-bladder, heart, and especially in the dynamics of the blood supply, we find the language of gesture in the corresponding vowels: 'I', 'O', 'E', 'Au'. The formative forces of the various vowels, which bring about different effects in the organs, are of a cosmic nature. We take them in through the air we breathe, since the air is always permeated by these cosmic formative forces. Should one of these organs be deformed, we can strengthen the healthy formative forces by vowel exercises and so work on the circulation through the breathing, right into the structure of the organ, but always by means of the rhythmic system. In the Curative Eurythmy Course we find this passage: 'We could also be dealing with faulty, objective inspiration which is expressed—if I may say so—in malformation of the rhythmic system. This deformation is made manifest particularly through the objective inspiration which, as it goes in, does not meet the circulation of the blood in the right way. Thus, when vowel eurythmy is used it has a normalizing effect.'

Every vowel exercise shows in its construction sound, limb-movement, hearing the sound again in inner calm, so that the vowel is made effective by way of the breath as it is inhaled (see Chapter 3).

It is important to hold fast to the idea that we can work on the deformity of the rhythmic system through the vowels. If there is severe deformity of an organ or deformity of the joints, consonants must be used first.

In speech the human being expresses, through the vowel sounds, his innermost being and experiences. We can always give vowels in curative eurythmy when we want to strengthen the ego within the sheaths. We can work discriminatively through the vowels in the prevailing conditions of warmth and air. Ego and astral body unfold their activity in these elements. One side of the vowel effect is the following: 'The distribution, the differentiation of the warmth conditions and air conditions play a large part in everything that has to do with forming and shaping.'

The vowel activity pours inwards through the respiration and circulation to reach the various organs in the congruity between planetary spheres—organs—vowels, as we know. From the organs the vowels ray out through the whole being and are reflected back from the head. They unfold their moulding, formative forces in this reflection. Thus they act on the various stages of life, as for example, 'U' on the hardening tendencies, the 'dying life'; 'A' on the building-up, 'strengthening life'. We appeal to these forces reflecting back from the head when we want to bring a person into himself by means of vowel exercises. This is expressed in the second guiding principle of vowel therapy. In doing vowel eurythmy what happens is that 'in the human being his own aura is drawn together to some extent, it is intensified in itself; this indeed is always the case in spiritual activity, and in this way the inner organs are stimulated to bring the human being into himself.'

When there is too much vowel activity in a person, when he experiences his inner being too strongly and does not relate himself sufficiently to what is around him, then he becomes an egoist organically. The organs themselves then lose their liquid-flowing growth forces and tend to become rigid and crystalline. 'Stomach and liver and the lobes of the lungs are actually in danger of becoming wedge-shaped. In this case the consonants, not the vowels, should be done in eurythmy. The vowel element is used when a person is as it were flowing out of himself organically.

We appeal to the reflection of the vowels from the head if we want to work on the formation of specific tissue structure—bones, muscles, cartilage, nerves. We shall see in our study of the consonants how our supersensible form is created from the forces of the zodiac (see Chapter 10). It is thanks to the planetary forces that this form is replete with substances which enable the human being to stand and walk on the earth and to perceive his surroundings. How 'A'-'O'-'U' influence the formation of bone, cartilage and muscle is described by J. Bort in the article '*Das A O U M im Blutkreislauf des Menschen*'. (Not translated.)

The knowledge of cosmic descent was given to man as a revelation; it came to him from outside. Since the Mystery of Golgotha a change has taken place which only now is making its full demands on humanity—not to allow this ancient wisdom to get lost. Each individual human being has to find the inner way back to the beginnings of his cosmic existence by seeking for a wider spiritual background of the visible world of the physical senses.

The medical-therapeutical path to the starry worlds is by way of the inner organs. Some important knowledge of this subject was given in the lectures *True and False Paths in Spiritual Investigation* given at Torquay in 1924. A way of investigation is described which starts with a precise knowledge of the anatomy, physiology and pathology of the organs as we know them today in scientific research, but the ultimate aim of which is to approach the spiritual prototype of the organ. If one tries to penetrate into the organ with spiritual perception and to intensify it until it becomes an imaginative grasp of the organ, this perception again can expand into cosmic spheres, for example, there can be recognition of the liver in the Jupiter sphere. 'Because these organs manifest themselves in the spirit, it is not merely the earthly man who stands there, but man who embraces the cosmos.'

This is a path of investigation which Rudolf Steiner followed and which points to the future. Already it has given rise to the book *Fundamentals of Therapy: An Extension of the Art of Healing through Spiritual Knowledge*, written by Rudolf Steiner in collaboration with Ita Wegman.

But how do we find this path? We have to go back to the very beginning of the creation of the physical body—to the Saturn evolution of the earth. The Saturn warmth is still active in us in the warmth of our blood. We can speak of man as if he were a warm room, for the warmth body of man is enclosed in itself—it keeps its temperature constant, apart from certain variations during the day, in relation to the environment. However, it does show differences in the various organs, some being warmer and others cooler. For instance, the normal temperature of the liver is about 40°C, while the temperature of the blood is normally about 37°C.

In entering deeply into the differentiated warmth-organism one is taking the first steps on the path to the spiritual spheres out of which the physical, bodily organs were once created.

As an exercise to start with, Rudolf Steiner pointed the way with the words:

> You have to look everywhere for Saturn ... and one becomes aware that the forces of Saturn work in a special way in every organ. They work, for

instance, most strongly of all in the liver, comparatively feebly in the lungs and least strongly of all in the head. The human being bears within him, in his organs, images of spiritual, divine beings. The whole cosmos which in the Saturn sphere was once an enormous human being, now becomes evident as a gigantic, cosmic being, in that it appears as the culmination, the inner-organic product of generations of gods working together. [21 August 1924.]

PART 2

CHAPTER 8

Vowels and Consonants

In a performance of artistic eurythmy we listen to the spoken word and see the connections of word and sense made visible in the movements of eurythmy. Vowels and consonants work together, and according to which of the two elements is predominant it gives its character to the speech and to the performance. If outer events are to be interpreted, if external things are to be shown vividly, then the consonants will be predominant. A lyrical, musical poem is carried more by the vowel element. The vowels express inner experience and, therefore, give words that otherwise remain the same in their consonantal make-up a completely different inner shade of feeling, as, for instance, the words last, list, lost, lust. Artistic performance will always be at pains to present the difference between consonants and vowels.

In curative eurythmy we often make use of *only vowels* or *only consonants* in certain illnesses. This one-sidedness is often necessary in therapy. Therefore some knowledge of the physiological effect of the vowels and consonants pertains to the basic principles of curative eurythmy. Rudolf Steiner has shown us the physiological–therapeutical difference from various points of view.

We see from the study of the Curative Eurythmy Course, and also from daily practice, that *one* important area for the use of consonants lies in the process of consumption of food, digestion and excretion. Every consonant has its specific function, e.g. 'H' in the stomach, 'T' in the small intestine, just as the digestive juices appear in specific regions. The consonants imitate the external world in gesture; they are plastic sculptors and through them we can acquire insight into the plastic formative forces working within the stiff and rigid world. Within the *human being* they break down what is taken in from the external world as food. The consonants work 'in the human organism initially on that which comes from the inherent dynamics of the substances of the world' and 'in what is developed in the human organism in overcoming the inherent vitality of the external essence'. The food substance is consumed and then assimilated by the kidney and the liver–gall-bladder systems and diffused through the whole organism. It encounters other forces coming as rounding-off forces from the head and skin organization. Here is an extremely interesting interplay, something which, it could be said, leads to the innermost depths of the human organism. Indeed the formation of the organism can be directly imagined as rays emanating from the kidney–liver system; and they are met by the plastic, formative forces of the head system.

> From the liver–kidney system such emanations take place—of course, not only upwards, but in all directions. These emanations tend to work semi-radially, but everywhere they are blunted by the plastic forms coming to meet them from the head system. Thus we can understand the *form of the lungs* by imagining their shape to have been moulded by the liver–kidney system; but coming to meet these components are those from the head system which round them off. Indeed the entire human form comes into being if we imagine: radial formation from the kidney–liver system, rounding-off of the radial formation from the head system. [27 October 1922.]

These words were spoken by Rudolf Steiner to doctors on the day before the lecture on curative eurythmy was given in Stuttgart, where this point of view again plays a large part. It shows the way to achieve an insight into the working together of consonants and vowels in the whole organism and in each organ. For in those forces which come from the kidney–liver system, forming the organs plastically from within, the consonants are active. In vowel eurythmy we live in the formative rounding-off element coming from the head. As examples the exercises 'L–A' and 'L–O' are well-known.

In the description of the interaction of consonants and vowels, Rudolf Steiner again and again appeals to the artistic mood of the soul, through which the curative eurythmist, starting from the impulses of movement, can acquire a deeper insight into the human organism. He says: 'From this you can see . . . that everything depends upon understanding how in each single human organ there is a kind of centrifugal dynamic force [consonant demonstrated], which is plastically rounded from the outside by a dynamic force working inwards upon each human organ [vowel demonstrated], i.e., it is not quite centripetal but can be called similar.'

The centrifugal and centripetal forces are presented by Guenther Wachsmuth [*Earth and Man*] as a polarity of formative forces in the human organism as follows:

> From this polarization in the field of activity of the etheric body of man, it follows that, as far as the inner dynamics are concerned, in the basic structure the centripetal, concentrating, solidifying formative forces are centralized mainly in the head. This has two consequences. Firstly, because of the predominance of the centripetal formative forces in the head, it is here that

man cuts himself off most strongly from his surroundings and creates thereby the kernel of his own inner world, his self-consciousness. But the centripetal dynamic forces also work right down into the material structure; for the highest development of bone substance, the most intensive mineralization is to be seen in the head where the vital life processes meet the greatest resistance, so that they are forced to be active more in the lower region, in the metabolic pole of the human organism ... In the human head the centripetal structural principle of a closed-in sphere is dominant; in the limb system the centrifugal tendency to radiate outwards predominates.

In the skull formation of the head, substance is denser, more concentrated, mineralized; in the lower part of man it is lighter, more flexible, enlivened. In the same way the ossifying process goes out from the head where the centripetal, compacting formative forces predominate; the vitalizing process goes out from the lower part of man where the centrifugal, loosening, radiating formative forces predominate.

These two processes can be followed right down into the inner activity of the organs and are demonstrated in the alternation of the centrifugal secretory phase with the centripetal assimilatory phase of the daily rhythm.

In this description there is much to be found that is already familiar from the effect of the vowels and consonants. At the same time we have to take into consideration that Dr Wachsmuth has represented the polarity of centrifugal and centripetal forces as being in the etheric body itself and is the result of the differentiation of the etheric body into warmth ether, light ether, chemical ether and life ether, whereby the life and chemical ethers form the centripetal pole in this sense, and the warmth and light ethers the centrifugal pole.

In the effects of vowels and consonants we have to take into consideration the activity of the higher members of the human being. This also solves the difficulty of the vowels working in the centripetal dynamic force through warmth and air. In the Curative Eurythmy Course we are told that it is particularly important for the effectiveness of the vowels to differentiate the warmth and air conditions in the organs. Neither do they work directly from the head; they work through the rhythmic system in man, and only achieve the full centripetal effect in their reflection back from the head. The actual words about the effect of the vowels are: 'the plastic rounding-off is effected by a dynamic force working from outside inwards, that is, not *quite* centripetal, but a *similar* dynamic force tending towards the centre.'

In doing vowel eurythmy we strengthen the actual human being, his inner self, the ego, in its relationship to the soul and also physiologically. This has two consequences: in the realm of the soul, tendencies towards instability are attacked; organically, the forces of form and figure are strengthened and the out-flowing of the organs is opposed. An individuality who is too shut up in himself can have these characteristics to an exaggerated degree; this leads him to become an egoist in his soul and the organs become over-formed, crystalline, wedge-shaped.

To overcome this tendency we use the consonants with their centrifugal, loosening, vitalizing, dynamic force. In doing consonantal eurythmy the human being places himself into the outer world, integrates himself in the being of the exterior world.

To summarize what has already been said—

Consonants are used:
> to stimulate all living processes, to relax the organism and make it more flexible in itself, to loosen any stiffness, to oppose obduracy in the soul and in the organs;
> to support in particular the digestive process in the manner already described;
> to improve any deformities already present and to try to reintroduce them into the formative process. Then when this has been achieved, we can use the vowels and so influence the right formation. Otherwise, by using the vowels the deformity could be worsened.

Vowels are used:
> to strengthen the formative forces, e.g. when an organ starts to become deformed;
> to stimulate the process of mineralization, e.g. 'A' and 'O' for teeth formation, 'U' for improving the bone structure;
> to strengthen the being itself, both emotionally and organically, e.g. 'I', to bring a person more strongly into himself.

*

To this list we must add that, as far as breathing is concerned, inhalation is activated by the consonants, exhalation by the vowels. In the breathing the polaric forces are balanced out. The digestive pole works in the breathing-in, the head pole in the breathing-out. Thus we see in the breathing not only a process of the lungs but a participation of the whole being.

If disorders appear in the breathing-in, e.g. shortness of breath, as often happens in illnesses of the kidneys, we can regulate it through the digestion with consonantal curative eurythmy. In disturbances of the breathing-out, e.g. in bronchial asthma, we try to help with vowel curative eurythmy. In the separate consonants we have a whole scale of different effects upon inhalation, from very strongly activating 'L' to 'M' and 'F' which influence exhalation as well. It is the same with the vowels, 'A' (ah) influencing inhalation, 'U' helping exhalation most. These will be dealt with in greater detail in the description of the various sounds.

This knowledge which has been given to us about the effect of the vowels and consonants on the breathing, whereby the whole human being is involved, makes it possible to create an enormous number of exercises for the regulation of the breath, according to how we put them together. Of course it goes without saying that the natural sequence of vowels and consonants in artistic eurythmy has a harmonizing effect on the whole human being and makes him into a better 'breather'.

*

Two further aspects of the effects of the vowels and consonants will be mentioned here without going into more detail. In a lecture given at Penmaenmawr [28 August 1923], Rudolf Steiner describes antimony as a medicine, and contrasts the forces of antimony with the albumenizing forces. At the end it is stated 'the vowel movements are used so that those forces which I just now called "albuminizing" forces in man are strengthened, whereas through the consonantal forces it is frequently the forces of antimony which are strengthened'. And so a balance can be established between these two forces through the co-operation of consonants and vowels in curative eurythmy.

In the Christmas course for doctors [January 1924], Rudolf Steiner speaks about the significance for man of the cosmic forces, and says:

> What heals in curative eurythmy is, basically—I would say—that which, in healing, depends most especially upon cosmic forces. When you do consonantal curative eurythmy exercises then you are in the Moon forces. When you develop vowel curative eurythmy forces, then you are in the Saturn forces. And through these two kinds of forces the human being feels himself drawn into the cosmos when he is doing curative eurythmy. To take an example: it might be possible to diagnose the following—for surely, in medicine, the main thing is the therapy but there can be no therapy unless there is first a useful diagnosis—but let us suppose that the diagnosis shows that the formative process in a person is too strong, so that, let us say, he has an excess of mineral salts or carbohydrates in him which he cannot overcome. [What is meant here is an excess of non-human formative substance. Ed.] If you really weigh up the finer effects of the organism—the symptoms could appear as only very slight indications—then vowel eurythmy, which works against the formative process, could have a very beneficial effect. Or again, let us suppose a small child shows a slight tendency to stutter. Now, of course, I do not wish to speak superficially and say that stuttering is caused by this or that; naturally, it could be the result of any one of a number of weaknesses, but in any case the damage has the effect of producing a predominant amount of formative force and, for this very reason, vowel curative eurythmy exercises are done for stuttering, and particularly in that

sequence which brings about a truly human manifestation of the vowel nature of man. It should be applied especially in this way. So that, in fact, if one has the necessary perseverance and zeal, a great deal may be achieved with children who have a tendency to stutter by simply using the ordinary curative eurythmy sequence of 'A E I O U'.

*

When the consonantal and vowel effects are put together in this rather theoretical way, one-sidedness cannot always be avoided. In actually working with patients the situation has to be kept alive and fluid by constantly keeping it in view.

So far we have described the consonantal effect in the digestion, whence it goes out to the blood circulation and breathing. If we study the consonants in their cosmic aspect, originating in the sphere of the zodiac, then they show us how they participate in the building-up of the human form. From the form of the head down to the creation of the feet, we can see how the figure is formed out of the forces of the zodiac (see Chapter 10). These forces surround the human being throughout his whole life, like a sphere, or an aura, holding him together. If they relax, then the human being loses himself in the world around him with the result that changes in the figure take place—crippling, deformity. We know from practice, and from many indications given by Rudolf Steiner, that then consonantal eurythmy is appropriate. In the Curative Eurythmy Course it says: 'a person who does consonantal eurythmy has the tendency to create a kind of aura around himself, which then works back upon him and brings him out of this condition of being engulfed by the insubstantiality of the world'.

To conclude, let us once more recapitulate the sentences in the curative Eurythmy Course which have a bearing on the use of vowels and consonants, although they have already been mentioned in the text.

Vowels:
'The arrangement, the differentiation of the warmth conditions in the human organism and the organization of the air conditions have an important part to play in everything that is of a plastic nature.'

'In a person who is made to do vowel eurythmy the effect is that his aura is drawn together to a certain extent, it is condensed *into itself*, which of course is always the case in spiritual activity, and the inner organs are thereby stimulated to bring the human being into himself.'

Consonants:
'For everything which is of a centrifugal nature, of a radiating nature, a great part is played, firstly, by what is in the human organism that

comes from the inherent dynamics of the substances of the world, and by what is developed in the human organism in overcoming the inherent vitality of the external essence.'

'A person who does consonantal eurythmy has the tendency to create a kind of aura *around himself* which then works back upon him and brings him out of this condition of being engulfed by the insubstantiality of the world.'

CHAPTER 9

The Consonants

The particular fields of application for the consonants will now be considered in what follows.

The sound 'L'

In the Speech Eurythmy Course it is said about 'L': 'It is the formative force which overcomes the material.' We can imagine that 'L' is the creative formative force which does the moulding in the etheric body. Since the ether body permeates the whole watery element in the human body, so 'L' also is active everywhere in the organism where the watery element is creative. The human organism consists for the most part of water. The solid parts are taken up into it, dissolving and condensing again. They are subject to the physical laws of gravity. The etheric body is not subject to these physical laws, but belongs to the etheric world with its different principles. While the physical laws work in such a way that they stream out from the earth and strive to orientate everything according to gravity, the etheric forces stream in from every side of the universe, from the periphery. They are the forces of buoyancy and have to struggle with the forces of gravity. How could a plant grow unless the forces of the circumference lifted it out of gravity and allowed the sap to flow upwards, in opposition to gravity! The living form is created in the interaction between these two streams of forces.

The drop of water, transformed into a plant, combines below with the soil, with the solid, and is metamorphosed into a root which adapts itself to the earth and is drawn into the gravitational force. The stalk, and with it the leaves spreading out into the surroundings, lifts itself up in opposition to gravity, creating a balance between weight and lightness, bringing about a reconciliation between them. The plant opens its blossom upwards to the light, giving itself up in colour and perfume. The 'L' gesture is inclined to sympathize with what is happening here. When executing the 'L' movement one feels oneself in harmony with the forces working everywhere in Nature, streaming in from the periphery.

With these forces of buoyancy permeating our arms we plunge them consciously into the forces of gravity, hold them in balance with the in-streaming plastic, formative force, and raise them up in an opening movement. The movement is rounded all the time and remains in the water element, striving to retain its drop-like form through all its metamorphoses.

The substance of earthly material is transformed through etheric action in the interchange of these polar forces. Matter is withdrawn from the scope of physical forces and etheric formative forces can give it shape and form. Matter is overcome by creative power; we look into a living event.

Form-giving life takes hold of dead matter; this takes on a new form and is expelled again as lifeless from the living stream. We are looking into the world of creation and decay, the continual metamorphosis of transformation. This is how the plant form originates in Nature; in man, organs are created which have a plantlike character, e.g. the glands.

'L' unfolds its activity chiefly in the realm between the watery–etheric and physical–solid elements. It strengthens the peripheral forces and can make the activities of the organism which have fallen prey to the forces of gravity prone to the influences of the etheric organization again. It leads the physical–etheric processes right up to the point of assimilation by the astral, the breathing. This is shown in the upward, opening gesture of 'L'.

A wide field of application for 'L' is thus opened up.

In the Curative Eurythmy Course it is stated that the 'L'-movement works particularly strongly on 'the peristaltic action, the actual intestinal movement'. It is indicated that the movement of the limb-digestive organism has a regulating effect on the circulation and breathing.

'L' is performed with a jump in which the legs are apart and the knees held together (this is known as the X-jump). This exercise is carried out with either a forward or backward jump, but preferably not on the spot.

Since many of the consonant exercises are given for constipation and affect the intestinal movement, we have to ask ourselves: what is the particular effect of the 'L'-exercise? The food is liquefied in the whole digestive tract, from the mouth to the intestines. Again and again the pulpy food mass has digestive juices poured over it. With so-called oscillatory movements of the intestines which consist in moving the contents of the bowels rhythmically to and fro, the food pulp gets well mixed and saturated with the secretions. By means of this process, in which the substance is dissolved and the food increasingly loses its identity through the effect of fermentation by the digestive juices, resorption through the intestinal wall is made possible. This means, though, that at the same time the food is raised upwards by degrees into the etheric processes and is made fit to be taken up into the human etheric body. We are looking here into a process that is akin to potentization. Here, too, the hidden forces in the substance are gradually released and made effective through rhythmical dilution and agitation.

The specification for 'L' clearly leads us into the realms of 'L'-activity previously described. We work with the 'L'-exercise—

> Firstly: on the secretion of the juices themselves. Some people's mouths water at the very thought of a favourite dish; with others the mouth and tongue remain dry—a symptom which points to a deficiency in the secretion of digestive juices. In such cases it is usually the whole digestive process that is upset.
> Secondly: on a thorough blending of foodstuff through stimulation of the peristaltic action.
> Thirdly: on making better use of the foodstuff so that it is fully prepared for absorption into the etheric.

Since in constipation many of these processes have become inert, it is easy to understand the beneficial effect of the 'L'-exercise which gets everything going again.

In the process of food digestion we see, therefore, that 'L' is active right up to the moment when the food becomes etherized. As a supersensible organization of forces the etheric body needs oxygen in order to be physically effective. The oxygen is necessary so that the etherized food becomes *alive in an earthly way*. So the flow of food presses on through the blood stream to reach the breath in order that it can get oxygen. This process is assisted by 'L'. We shall be speaking further about the activation of the breathing process by means of 'L'.

The etheric body of man is something whole—a mobile organism, individual to each human being. It is the sculptor of the body and pervades the organism during life with formative forces of renewal and growth. The whole fluid human being is the bearer of the etheric activity. It is the blood, above all, that belongs properly to the fluid human being as it flows in a rhythmical stream from the heart to the periphery and back to the centre of the body. Tissue fluid, lymph, chyle, and the crystal-clear fluid washing around the brain and the spinal cord are all part of the fluid man.

In the tissue fluid, in the lymph, in fact wherever the watery element is unorganized and does not pulse in rhythmical movement, we must look for the interaction between what is living and what is lifeless. Many disorders can originate here. Substances can escape too soon from the flow of the stream of life; mineral deposits are formed; indeed, water which has been permeated with life but not by the breath, can bring about congestion and oedema in the tissues.

When the quickening, moving force of buoyancy is lacking, then heaviness can prevail even in the circulation—tiredness, a feeling of heaviness, sluggish circulation, can all occur.

Many years of experience have shown how helpful the 'L'-exercise can be for these symptoms when it is repeated often. Actually doing the exercise shows that we have to be particularly careful that the 'L', with its loosening and quickening powers, enters actively enough into the heaviness. A light, superficial 'L', done high up and without stressing the character sufficiently in arms and hands, can be disastrous. It can result in heaviness and buoyancy becoming still more widely separated. The 'L' is not always done with knock-knees, but it is a help when knees and body are moved together in the manner indicated by Rudolf Steiner in the Speech Eurythmy Course: 'In the fluid sound of "L" make the movement of the body itself an enthusiastic, rhythmical swing, forwards—backwards, forwards—backwards, so that you get it right down into the physical body.' If possible the rocking should be done with such intensity that one almost falls over forwards or backwards, but just manages to keep one's balance. This movement, which puts a great strain on the knees, strengthens the circulation of the blood. Unsteadiness and pain in the knees can often be an early sign of circulatory disorders.

The patient has to learn just as painstakingly to form the 'L'-movement, loosening and opening upwards, so that the etheric can be properly permeated by the breath.

This is especially important in cases of weeping eczema with enlarged tonsils and adenoids, a tendency to catarrh. Many children, and also different types of children, show a tendency to this kind of constitutional anomaly. Disorders of the lymphatic system are predominant. The etheric is not sufficiently accessible to the breathing. The characteristic facial expression of the child with overgrown adenoids in the nose and throat region is well known to all. Breathing and speech defects are the result of these excrescences. Sounds like 'M' and 'N' become blurred; 'P', 'T', 'K' are produced very indistinctly. The open mouth shows how difficult it is to breathe.

We use 'L' a great deal for such children by itself and also in sequences, such as 'L-M-S-U', or else 'L-M' alone, to strengthen the breathing. Reports on school work show again and again how frequently one has to deal with such children, and how much benefit they can derive from these exercises.

In most cases of obstructed breathing, short-windedness, asthma or adenoidal outgrowths, we start with 'L'. Together with 'M', which in its turn works strongly on exhalation, we have a very powerful exercise in the 'L-M' sequence for deepening and harmonizing the breathing.

*

But how shall we describe the abounding virtues of 'L', the soothing, relaxing strength of this movement, through which all stiffness in soul and body is loosened, and crippled limbs can gradually be made to move again?

'L' belongs to the etheric body, and the etheric body is the healer in man. We call upon the regenerative powers of the etheric body in all healing processes. So it is not surprising that with most patients we practise 'L' as well as other sounds. If we take the precautions already described, and see that the gesture is properly directed into the heaviness and towards the loosening, then there can be no risk of danger. Since at the present time people tend to be immobile and stiff in the etheric, the efficacy of remedies and other methods of healing can be enhanced through loosening and quickening the etheric with 'L'.

It is more difficult to understand that 'L' is sometimes approached as a formative force, sometimes as the formative substance in itself. In Nature we find an earthly substance, clay, silicate of argillaceous earth, which combines in itself the forming and formative forces as does 'L'. Clay, in its pure form, is used for making pottery and porcelain. It has the capacity to take on form and retain it and therefore it is used for modelling and making pottery. When it is moist it can be plastically shaped, when it is dry it can hold the shape it has been given. Clay is also a fertile soil; plants thrive in it. The middle part of the plant, the leaves, grows large and strong. Strong etheric life can unfold on this soil.

We feel something of this good, fruitful earth when we read in *Eurythmy as Visible Speech*: '"L" can be experienced as something real, as if one were to eat a dumpling that has a particularly good flavour, and because it is not hard, but rather soft, it melts in the mouth in a feeling of inner well-being.'

The living stream of substance in man is the plastic material. The formative forces, weaving in all living things, imprint the image of the organs into this plastic material. What are the forces that work as formative forces in the etheric body? We get the answer from the second lecture of the Curative Education Course:

> We are surrounded by the physical world. But also by the etheric world, from which, as you know, our own etheric body is taken immediately before we descend into physical incarnation. The etheric body of man comes from the cosmic ether, which is all around us everywhere. Now this cosmic ether, my dear friends, is in reality the bearer of thoughts. The cosmic ether, common to us all, carries the thoughts within it; there they are, those living thoughts of which I have repeatedly spoken in our anthroposophical lectures, telling you how the human being participates in them in pre-earthly existence,

before he comes down to earth. All such thoughts are contained there in a living way in the cosmic ether and are never taken from the cosmic ether during life between birth and death. Man's whole stock of living thought which he holds within him, he receives at the moment when he descends from the spiritual world, that is, when he leaves his own element of living thought, and descends to form his etheric body. The living thoughts are still there, within man, as forming and organizing forces. [26 April 1924.]

We know that during the first years of life after birth, the etheric body is entirely occupied with forming and organizing activity. After certain epochs—in the 7th, the 14th and the 21st years of life—these forces are no longer so tied up with the organic activity; they become free, they enable man to form thoughts. This process has been frequently described in anthroposophical educational literature. It is one of the basic ideas for the development of education and curative education.

We would only point out here that we try to help children who do not find it easy to learn or to develop their own thinking, with the sequence 'R-L-S-I' (see Chapter 12).

At his entry into life man has been creating out of the universal world-ether; and what he has brought with him in the way of etheric forces is a reservoir for his whole life. Much can be done from many aspects to keep these forces of the etheric body flexible and active and in communion with the world-ether, so that they do not become wooden and immobile.

The more we come to know the etheric body, the more alive does the healing power of the sound 'L' become.

The sound 'R'

Indications are given in the Curative Eurythmy Course for the 'R'-exercise:

1 'R' is something 'which regulates the evacuation rhythm when it is not in order'.
   In this case 'R' must be done for only a short time, a few minutes, but then several times a day.
2 An 'R', in which the trunk is moved vehemently, forwards and backwards in bending and stretching, 'works very well on the whole rhythmic system, especially on the breathing and circulatory rhythm'.

In 'R' we have a sound which unfolds its activity in the rhythmic man. It was shown in the first chapter how rhythm is connected with the involuted forces of the astral body. By creating an inside and an outside a rhythmical correlation springs up between the two. This rhythmical activity comes most fully into its own in the air-organism which is the bearer of the astral body. In the process of inhalation and exhalation it becomes clear how the air that is within us is in continual rapid interchange with the outer air, and through this with the atmospheric influences of light and warmth. The breathing rhythm meets the rhythm of the blood inside us and continues through the whole being in the blood. In every organ there is an exchange of air, an interchange of gas. The air-man is just as much a reality as the mineral and the watery-man.

The rhythmic activity of the breathing and circulation unites and harmonizes in man the great polarity of the digestive-limb system and the nerve-sense system and creates thereby a balance between the centripetal and the centrifugal processes. It is clearly perceptible that the centripetal forces are localized in the head. The world of the senses is outside, surrounding us. The sense impressions stream in from outside and are perceived from within. This whole process leads from the outer world to the inner world of the organism. The processes proceeding from the digestion are centrifugal. Substances are digested within but the activity and movement of the limbs is directed outwards, leading to the performance of actions and deeds in the world. Rudolf Steiner tells the curative eurythmist again and again to observe the centrifugal and centripetal processes, not only as they occur on a large scale but also in the finer processes of each single organ. The hardening, mineralizing processes originate in the centripetal forces of the head, the living, softening processes from the centrifugal processes (see Chapter 8).

'R' is the vibratory sound—the movement has to resemble an inner agitation, a trembling. From the shoulders into the hands, right into the fingertips, the vibrations of the sensitive air-man have to be rendered in movement. In the fingertips, where the movement meets the external element of air, it does not break off but vibrates back into itself. What is characteristic of all rhythmical processes is that they do not go on for ever, but turn rhythmically inwards upon themselves. Even when we do 'R' with forward and backward bending of the trunk—an exercise which we call the little rhythmical 'R'—the 'R' still has to remain a vibratory sound. It is difficult for the patient to learn, and one has to discern whether the inner activity and sensibility are being sufficiently stimulated, whether the air-man is being made to vibrate. The hands often remain like wilting leaves, just lying on the air, instead of becoming one with it. Then ways have to be found to make a proper 'R', so that the balance is held between going out with the air and turning back into oneself, between surrender and self-assertion. With this rhythmical 'R', which is considered to be one of the soul-exercises, we can work prophylactically, as long as there is no question of any serious organic disorder in the rhythmic system, but instability in the soul shows that slight irregularities of the rhythmic system are already beginning.

For obvious illnesses, for shortness of breath, bronchial or cardiac asthma, we begin with exercises like: 'Yes—No', 'L–M', 'L–A–O–U–M', and lead on gradually to the 'R'-exercise, because 'R' is too hard at first and can be too much of an intrusion.

If we want to work on the evacuation rhythm with 'R', then we do the curative eurythmy 'R' with the whole body; we call it the big 'R'. We commence the 'R' with arms and legs while making a step either forwards or backwards with bent knees. The rotating, rounding movement of 'R' must involve the whole body. In straightening up again the vibrating movement must also be felt along the entire length of the spinal column.

As already mentioned, the exercise is done only for short periods at a time, but three or four times a day. Where there is a tendency to severe constipation it has a strong and rapid effect. With this exercise the astral body is stimulated into active movement. In describing the exercise Rudolf Steiner begins with the leg movement and lays great stress on the stepping forwards, and the bending and stretching of the legs. It is not a matter of indifference whether we emphasize the arm or the leg movement in an exercise. For the point about the intervention of the astral is the difference between arms and legs. Man's arms are not incorporated in gravity; we move our hands and arms about freely and through them have the possibility of free creation. The legs, though, are entirely restricted by gravity. This is caused by the different kind of connection of the astral body with the arms and legs. The astral body has a much looser connection with the arms than with the legs. In massage this fact is taken very much into consideration. It is known that massage of the arms and hands affects more the *inner* digestion, as far as the formation of the blood, while massaging the legs and feet has more to do with that part of the digestion which is connected with evacuation and excretion. This is also important for curative eurythmy. The big 'R' can be further assisted by doing 'R' with the legs only, either sitting or standing: this exercise is also given for fat people. It works particularly on excretion. But if one wants to regulate the digestion as far as the circulation, then 'R' should be done mostly with the arms.

Can we also affect the rhythms of the head organization with 'R' as we affect the evacuation rhythms in the digestion? Our attention is directed to three very different 'Rs': the 'Labial-R', which is expressed in the movement by forming the 'R' low down; the 'Tongue-R', formed in the horizontal; the 'Palate-R', which is done high up.

An important explanation given by Rudolf Steiner of the rhythmical principle in the head organization can be quoted here:

In our head organization we have a rhythmical life. Sometimes we are more inclined to respond from within to sense perceptions, at other times are are less disposed to react to them; it is just that these changing conditions span a period of 24 hours. And it would be interesting, perhaps by means of graphs, to observe how people differ in respect of this inner head rhythm, alternating between bright, animated powers of conception and dull, sleepy ones. For the dull, sleepy conceptual powers are, as it were, an inner night of the head; while the bright ones are an inner day time of the head. This does not coincide with the external rhythm of day and night. There is an inner alternation between lightness and darkness. And according to whether a person tends more to have this inner rhythm between light and dark so that the light part, when his conceptual powers are bright, coincides with his sense perceptions, or whether the dark part coincides with his sense perceptions, according to whether the one or the other is in a person's organization, he differs in his potentiality, his faculty, for observing the external world. The one has a strong propensity to observe outer phenomena closely, while the other is less disposed to observe external phenomena closely; he turns more to inner brooding. This is precisely the result of what I have just been describing. Especially as educators, we should accustom ourselves to making such observations, for they give us important hints on how to deal competently with children in their up-bringing and education. [8 January 1921.]

We have not, however, as yet, enough experience to establish whether doing the 'R' low down is particularly effective in cases where it is desired to influence the head rhythm.

*

The great rhythm of sleeping and waking is important for a healthy life. On waking, the ego and astral body re-enter the etheric and physical body from which they withdraw on going to sleep. It is a great respiration which takes place chiefly between the etheric body and the astral body. 'R' is not used a great deal as an actual exercise for insomnia, but there are accompanying symptoms of defective going to sleep or waking up which can often be tackled only with 'R'. Going to sleep is made more difficult when the astral body does not easily free itself from the etheric. This adherence of the astral body to the physical–etheric body can lead to various symptoms which are not at first connected with the process of sleeping and waking. Rudolf Steiner has pointed out that some disturbances of movement are accompanying symptoms of not being able to go to sleep properly; such things as every involuntary twitch of the eyes, too much bending of the fingers, all fidgety movements of the body, indeed any movement that is not the expression of an inner process. All eurythmy which, as such, gives external expression of gesture again to the inner processes will be of help here.

Special 'R' is used with good results when the forces of the astral body have been over-strained and have led to occupational neuroses. These are usually caused by certain groups of muscles being used too much and too one-sidedly, mostly in fine and intricate occupations. The best known is writer's cramp, the cramp which violinists or cello players get, and the dentist's cramp in the right hand. It is often difficult to control these troublesome complaints therapeutically; and it is therefore gratifying to have an effective aid in 'R'.

The general accompanying symptoms of defective waking are better known: inertia, numbness, dullness, even disturbed consciousness.

'R' can help in both directions to compensate and regulate rhythm. If it has once been recognized that 'R' can assist the dipping in and out in all rhythmical processes, then it can also be readily understood that the eurythmy figure for 'R' has green for the character. In the spectacle of the rainbow, green lies in the middle, between red on the one hand and blue on the other, at the turning-point, as it were, where what went in is beginning to come out again.

In discussions on curative eurythmy the question has sometimes emerged whether we should not give more consideration to the individual rhythms of organs. Modern research into rhythm can give us a foundation here. Guenther Wachsmuth points out the rhythmical functions of the various organs, liver, kidneys, which are partly conditioned by the activity of the organs themselves and partly depend on the geological and cosmological conditions. Studying this book gives us a fundamental insight into the rhythmical phases of centripetal and centrifugal processes of individual organs.

Experience in this field of curative eurythmy is not yet available. It will certainly be necessary to go more deeply into this question to work out a ratio as to whether one should differentiate between the daily or the weekly rhythm of the individual organs.

The sound 'S'

When we occupy ourselves with the sound 'S' there is one picture which we can hold before our mind's eye. It is the picture of the staff of Mercury which was so impressively presented in the carved pillars of the old Goetheanum. The architrave over the fourth pillar shows the staff of Mercury with *two* pillars and two serpents which, in the capital of the fifth column, are harmoniously united into *one* staff intertwined by two serpents. Only to look at them fills us with invigorating peace. Much of the effectiveness of the sound 'S' in the human organism can become clear to us through this picture; it can help us to get through to what is essential in the sound, so that 'S', with its great healing power, can become ever more and more effective.

Some words of Rudolf Steiner may be quoted here which make the connection between the 'S'-sound and Mercury's staff clear: 'It could be said that the experience of the 'S'-sound is connected with what was experienced at the beginning of human evolution in the snake symbol, or in a certain sense, what was felt about the symbol of the mercurial staff—not for the actual symbol of Mercury itself, but for the symbol of Mercury's *staff*.'

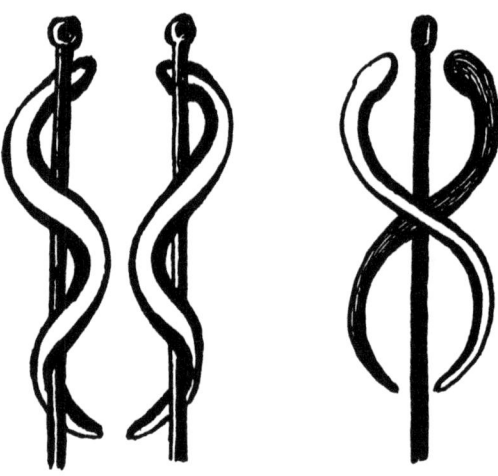

In our script 'S' has the form of a snake. In eurythmy, too, the S-gesture is a snake-like movement. The first information Rudolf Steiner gave about 'S' was: 'Comply to form.' The snake-like movement is formed with the hands and arms and one is putting oneself thereby into the outer formative power of 'S'; the movement goes on through the hands and arms into the whole body. We like to do 'S' with a rod or a veil to indicate 'giving form from outside'. Since the exercise is not easy to learn, it is often done at first with one arm, left and right alternately. But ultimately one must get to doing the movement with both arms simultaneously. Rudolf Steiner's brief remark that the power of 'S' to avert something with control lies precisely in the relationship *between* the arms is made clear to us in the above picture.

What is it that has to be averted with control by the S-movement? In the picture there are two snakes. The snake is the symbol for the old, instinctive wisdom which was given to man at a time when he was not endowed with an ego. In olden times this instinctive wisdom worked in a right way. It lives on in the animal. Through his ability to stand upright and through the development of his brain which makes it possible to think clearly, man has overcome the animal instincts. While in the animal the outer configuration and also the inner form of the organs are formed entirely by the astral body, in man the configuration is arrested by the astral body and both the inner and outer configuration is subject to the human ego-organization. But in the lower part of man there is continually a tendency, an inclination, to become animal again, and some symptoms of an illness show that the patient is too much disposed to take into himself again, as organic animal processes, the animalism which in the course of his development he has cast aside. Flatulence, eructation, a tendency to form haemorrhoids, putrid diarrhoea, all point to such processes.

As a curative eurythmy remedy against these symptoms we use 'S', 'for the "S"-movement works especially on the regulation of gaseous formations in the intestines. When this process is not in order, when it is either too inactive or too active, the "S"-movement will be found to be eminently successful'. The animal nature, or rather let us call it the lower astral nature of man, has to work to a certain degree in the lower organism. The digestive processes, indeed, all that has to do with the digestion of food, and above all what is connected with evacuation, both from the bowels and from the kidneys, all this comes under the control of the astral forces. When the astral body works too strongly on its own in these parts, then there is a tendency to neglect the excretions and to allow animal formative forces to develop. A characteristic sign of this is the formation of gases in which the air bubbles are trying to take on form and become an organ. Very often the formation of flatulence is connected with an inner organic disturbance and with agitation. These disturbances in the digestion which do not come from disquietude of the mind nor result in fidgeting of the limbs are due to an astral uneasiness in the region which is dependent on the vegetative, sympathetic nervous system. It continues beyond the digestion into the bloodstream and reaches the heart where it causes feelings of anxiety which oppress the heart with dull fears for life and limb, and can lead on to organic disturbances such as palpitations of the heart, shortness of breath, high blood pressure. This organic disorder can even express itself in dreams; dreams of wild animals and threatening situations can occur.

The power of the ego is lacking in the digestive system which can control these disorders and 'divert them by mastering them'. This power is strengthened by 'S'. The astral uneasiness is pacified, the activity of the astral body is included once more in the proper movement of the intestines and the spurious formations thereby dispelled. 'S' brings into the organism formative powers which are associated with the ego. The bad dreams then also disappear.

There are several examples of this to be taken from the consulting room. There was a woman who suffered a great deal from dreams of wild animals, but after she had been doing 'S' for a time she felt a change taking place. In the end she dreamt that she was taking a little pig for a walk on a lead. After that she was never again afflicted with the other kind of dream.

A patient with digestive disorders dreamt frequently of animals, especially of snakes which distressed him so deeply that he suffered great anguish. After he had been practising 'S' for some time, he dreamt one night of a python which was coming towards him. But he was no longer afraid because he was himself holding a small snake in his hand and with this he could subdue the large one.

*

Let us return once more to the staff of Mercury. In the staff itself we see the symbol of ego-organization, in the two snakes right and left, the animalistic forces which have been subdued. Rudolf Steiner's words come alive. 'The "S"-sound has always been of very great importance, even in the Mystery Schools. Indeed, even magical powers were, in fact, attributed to it. For it can be felt to have a soothing effect on something, and carries with it a feeling of assurance that the "S"-sound is capable of bringing peace and calm into what is in a state of turmoil by penetrating into the hidden nature of a being.' [18 April 1921.] This calming effect of 'S' enters right into the inner processes of man's life. When symbols full of wisdom from an ancient state of consciousness were given, they expressed actual processes within the human being, which could be regarded as etheric streams. Rudolf Steiner mentions the origin of Mercury's staff in connection with the radiating processes of various metals. The forces which have to be effective in the lower part of man and which work outwards from the intestinal tract in the excreta, and also all that is connected with the sexual processes, these forces take their course in man like the staff of Mercury.

Thus 'S' works right into the inner being, tranquillizing unconscious instincts in the organic process, warding off trouble in the bloodstream, reconciling sympathy and antipathy. The soothing power of 'S' has always been recognized. Even today one says 'Ssss' to reduce noise in a room. Restless children are quietened if one only feels inside oneself the inner attitude of 'S'.

*

'S' is a sibilant sound. We need the whole fire of our will to form it. At the same time an account must be given of the powerful formative forces contained in 'S'. Just as a diamond, as the hardest stone, is also the most fiery, so the 'S'-gesture combines within itself formative ability and controlled fire. The 'S'-form shows itself in many ways in the organism: in motion, in the peristaltic action of the small intestine; when it becomes fixed in the convolutions of the brain and in the bony structure it is stamped into the formation of the spinal column. Because of its strong, formative ability, 'S' also has a hardening, ossifying effect.

This can make clear to us what Rudolf Steiner says in the Curative Eurythmy Course, namely, that 'S' is really the ahrimanic sound which is also expressed in the grey, black and brown of the eurythmy figure. Movement goes over into fixation, is cast in a mould, and therein lies the ahrimanic element of 'S'. Since 'S' also bears inner fire within it, it has also the power to dissolve again that which has become solid. Therefore we can use 'S' for stony formations in the gall-bladder and kidneys. In therapy, therefore, one must always have in mind the double power of 'S'.

We have seen how in the lower part of man, when the animal processes take the upper hand, this can lead to symptoms such as gastric cramp, colics, diarrhoea, a tendency to haemorrhoids, period pains and cessation of the period, etc. In the upper part of man it is reflected as dullness, confusion and headaches. The light process in the upper man, which is the basis for thinking, cannot take place when the tendency to animal processes in the lower man gains the upper hand through not meeting with any resistance.

The knowledge that 'S' works as a regulator when there is either too much or not enough gas developed in the intestine gives rise repeatedly to the question: what is to be understood by *not enough* gas formation? The air element is connected, as we know, with the astral. The astral body is active wherever air appears in the organism. But if the astral body is not sufficiently involved in the digestion of the earthly substances in the activity of the lower organism this can bring about the unhealthy condition of insufficient gas being formed. Just as when there is too little etheric activity in the digestion not enough digestive juices are secreted, so it is when the astral body does not enter sufficiently into the element of air. It does not develop any tendencies of form, but neither does any movement arise. The intestinal peristalsis can become so inert that it comes to a standstill, becomes paralysed.

*

The curative eurythmy 'S' is connected with an 'O'-jump with the legs forwards and backwards. If the patient is not able to do the jump, then he should at least try to form the 'O' with his legs, either standing still or walking.

'S' is included in many of the sequence exercises and will be discussed then. Again and again we see its dual character: activating and soothing, fiery and formative, e.g. in the sequence of 'S-U-L-A' which is used for stunted growth. The child who for the first time was given the exercises had the typical old-man look of a dwarf. When maturity is attained too early the growth processes are suppressed. First the abnormal forming process is broken down and transformed by 'S', then growth is stimulated by 'L-A'.

'S' is very characteristic in the exercise 'L-M-S' used for goitre. In this illness we are dealing with a stiffening of the astral body. Digestive trouble, too much digestive activity, is very pronounced. Because of its stiffness the astral body does not allow the ego-organization to be active enough organically. The prominent eyeballs show that the formative forces coming from outside are lacking.

In the Curative Education Course Rudolf Steiner gave the case history of an illness which is very significant for the study of the sound 'S'. It concerns a 10-year-old girl who was retarded in her intellectual development owing to growths in the nose-throat area, and therefore had special difficulty in memory formation. As a result of spiritual investigation Rudolf Steiner found that these physical growths in the nose-throat area were like a mirror picture of excessive etheric growth in the region of the bladder. The interaction between the etheric body and the astral body could not take place properly and therefore the etheric body was forming excessive growth in the bladder region and was not properly connected in this part with the physical body. For this reason the child was unable to assimilate impressions sufficiently, nor could she inwardly digest and retain them as memories.

> For consider how it is with memory. Memory is dependent on a right and proper organic relationship between physical body and etheric body. Astral body and ego have no part in what is retained as impressions in memory. Dreams make their appearance only when the astral body and ego have begun to enter into the physical and etheric body, not before. As far as astral body and ego are concerned, everything is forgotten between the times of falling asleep and awakening. The impressions are left lying in the part of the human being that remains in the bed. But when, as in the child we are considering, this part is not properly organized, then what is left there of the impressions of the day does not combine with the body, and it will be a question, first of all, of awakening strong impressions in the mind in order to make the upper organization actively effective in the lower organization; I mean the ego and astral body in the etheric body and physical body. [6 July 1924.]

On the educational side one tried through rhythmical exercises to strengthen the ability to take in impressions.

Therapeutically, compresses of *Berberis vulgaris* were made to reduce the physical growths in the neck.

As a curative eurythmy exercise, 'L–M–S–U' was used and the following observed:

> You see, here again there is the underlying idea that the formative, clinging quality comes into the movement of the astral body to meet the 'M'. As I have already told you, 'M' is what puts the whole organism into exhalation, so that thereby, the astral and etheric organization can come together. 'S' is there in order to set the astral body in vigorous, vital activity, but in such a way that it restrains itself, and that is the purpose of the 'U'. [6 July 1924.]

The sounds 'H' and 'Sch'

According to the Curative Eurythmy Course, 'H' is used to 'regulate bowel activity in the region where the stomach passes into the intestine'. 'Sch', it is said, has a special effect 'on the stomach, on those parts at the beginning of the intestinal organism'. 'A weak digestion', so that 'the food remains in the stomach', is a sign that this sound should be used. Besides this it draws attention to the acidity in the stomach.

Digestive processes differ in the various sections of the intestines. First the food is broken down mechanically in the mouth. The digestion of carbohydrates is started by the ferment in the saliva, ptyalin. The digestion of protein starts in the stomach, as also does a part of the digestion of fats. However, the main part of the digestion of fats takes place in the small intestines.

In the mouth we become aware of the process of taste. As in all conscious sense-perception this is an activity of ego-organization. The real ego activity, through which we perceive the quality of our food, is often overlaid by sympathy and antipathy towards certain substances; this is where the astral body comes in.

In the stomach the digestion of food comes completely under the influence of the astral body. Indeed, the tasting process continues throughout the whole digestion. Each organ selects by taste the substance it needs from the food proffered. Thus it is that, although there is sufficient food, if the diet is unbalanced some organs can be starved, while others are overfed. In the stomach this tasting process takes place further, but it is no longer perceptible to our consciousness. What the ego does is now overlaid by the activity of the astral body which determines the digestion in the stomach. This is shown to be so from the physiological–chemical processes of the stomach. Wherever acidity appears in the organism, there the astral body has the controlling activity. The stomach is the only organ in which free acidity appears. Free hydrochloric acid is necessary for the functioning of pepsin which can only take place in an acid reaction. After a heavy meal the stomach secretes about 1 litre (1¾ pints) of gastric juice. At the same time a great deal of acidity is formed. Then the acidity in the rest of the organism begins to diminish and the alkalinity is increased. The acid–base economy in the body is to be regarded as a whole, and the fluctuations of acid and base reflect, as in a mirror, the interplay between astral body and ether body.

On the one hand the activity of the astral body is to be seen in the free hydrochloric acid. On the other hand, we have a permanent bubble of air in the stomach; here, too, we can see the close relationship between the stomach and the astral body. In more recent research this air bubble is supposed to influence the movement of the stomach—but it is seen purely as a mechanical effect depending on pressure from the diaphragm.

We must accustom ourselves to regarding the higher members of the human being as driving forces. This shows us more than ever how complicated the human organism is. It is not enough to have some general knowledge of the higher members. In each organ or organ region they are differently connected with each other and are active in a different reciprocal relationship. An organ is healthy when for this particular organ there is just the right blending of the activities of ego, astral body and etheric body. In the stomach region the astral body is not so closely connected with the ego-organization as it is in the rhythmical system; it adapts itself to the etheric body, but is rhythmically active by virtue of its own power. The way in which the sounds 'H' and 'Sch' are done in curative eurythmy must take into account this rhythmical incidence. Both are done slowly, with pauses, and 'Sch' indeed with a definite rhythm. 'H' is accompanied by a jump which is intrinsic to the 'H'-gesture. To begin the jump we stand with legs together, and only as we jump forwards do we spread out the legs and keep them apart as we come to a halt. After each jump there is a longish pause in which one can count up to 5 or 7. During the pause, the stimulus which has just been given should be allowed to take its effect. 'Sch' is accompanied by a number of jumps which are rhythmically articulated, thus: short–long–short–pause; long–short–long–pause; short–long–short–pause; and so on. 'Sch' is formed with every jump.

In speech, 'H' is like a puff of wind, on which we would like to stream out altogether. As a eurythmic sound-movement, 'H' has the same effect; we want to free ourselves from the organism and flow out into the element of light. A severe jolt is necessary to achieve this in movement.

So the 'H' gesture is a powerful movement going out from the shoulders and flinging both arms wide apart. The significant thing about this is that we experience this movement as consonantal, as something brought about from without, as an imitation of how the air drifts towards us in the process of breathing, which is why we open ourselves wide in this gesture.

To understand the effect of the sound 'H' on the human organism, we turn first of all to the exercise of 'eurythmic laughter'. This exercise shows in a more concentrated way what happens in the human being as a whole when he laughs. Our soul liberates itself in laughter, sets itself above the distressing things of life. For our astral body this means an expansion of itself, a broadening out, even a *relaxation*. Tensions are relieved. Even in the most tragic circumstance it can happen that someone bursts out laughing because he thereby releases the tension. In weeping the astral body contracts. Laughing and weeping signify an intensification of our breathing. Laughter, as we all know, acts on inhalation, it brings about a short breath out and a long breath in. 'There is a relaxation of the astral body in the process of laughing. It is just as if you were to pump all the air out of some space, rarefy the air: the air then comes hissing in. It is the same with the long indrawn breath under the influence of laughter . . . Whenever there is laughter the ego brings about an expansion, a broadening, a bulging of the astral body.' [27 April 1909.] We realize this in the 'H' gesture—expansion, liberation of oneself takes place.

The two aspects of 'H' show the effect on the breathing, the opening out and taking into oneself of all the light and formative forces that stream into us with the air we breathe. This effect can be clearly distinguished, for instance, against the activity of 'R' which also works on the breathing. 'R' is in itself a weaving rhythm of breathing in and out. 'H' lives in greater contrasts; it wants to lift the astral body out of the organic activity. Rudolf Steiner speaks about the luciferic character of 'H'. This stands in opposition to the surprisingly firm attitude which is presented in the eurythmy figure for 'H'. There the whole figure is in an attitude of self-confidence which is especially marked in the firmness with which the heels are set on the ground.

If one sees patients who need the 'H' exercise, it is striking how little movement there is in the thorax and how irregular is the inbreathing and outbreathing. Occasionally a deep breath is taken, but generally the breathing is shallow and weak. The front part of the chest is stiff and rigid and as if it were in a state of continual in-breathing; there is no proper opening-out, with the result that the breath is exhaled jerkily. Irritations of the larynx, nervous clearing of the throat, difficulty in swallowing, can all be connected with this condition. The astral body cannot relax. The condition can best be described in the words: the human being cannot 'let go of himself'. 'The 'H'-gesture shows us exactly how to let go, which, in the exercise, should not go too far and into the luciferic, but rather it must be controlled by the ego. In the exercise of 'eurythmic laughter', 'H' is followed by forming an 'A'. This should always be done in a downward direction which also prevents too much relaxation.

In contrast to 'H', 'Sch' has more power of contracting, bringing everything into brisk movement. We need only remind ourselves of the example Rudolf Steiner chose for 'Sch', Husch-husch, whereby 'Sch' represents what is 'blown away', that is, a sound gesture containing something which leads on, sets something in motion.

*

Let us now return to the effect of 'H' and 'Sch' in the stomach region. We shall have to look for disorders in this region corresponding to the relatively free, direct action of the astral body in the motility as also in the acidity conditions. Both can vary in two ways. In the *movement* of the stomach these disorders lie in a tendency to cramp conditions, or in a tendency to atony, the gradual relaxation or debility of the stomach muscles. Also in the formation of acid we have a pendulum, swinging between too much and too little. Superacidity, as well as subacidity and anacidity, are frequent symptoms of illness and have a bad effect on the organism as a whole. Intensified stomach movements are observed in secretory disorders, when the secretion of hydrochloric acid is either excessive or insufficient. They occur also when there is an obstruction in the outlet from the stomach which can be caused either functionally (pylorospasmus) or mechanically (constriction, due to local processes of illness = stenosis). In this case, however, relaxation soon follows the increased activity.

Nervous agitation can also stimulate increased peristaltic movements of the stomach even without organic cause. Since the activity of the stomach lies predominantly under the influence of the astral body, the stomach is, therefore, a sensitive organ reflecting the fluctuations of the soul-life. Everyone knows how unexpected excitement or a shock can 'go to the stomach', as the popular phrase has it. Experiences in the soul trigger off intense organic reaction in the epigastric region. In excitement or shock the astral body thrusts itself directly into the physical body—without the mediation of the etheric body—and is expressed as pain and also by increased secretory activity. If a person is continually exposed to too much agitation, or overwork, or finds himself in situations of emotional conflict, then stomach illnesses can develop on grounds of so-called nervous disorders. When the astral body intrudes too often and too intensively in the organic processes, this ultimately has a deleterious effect. It results in inflammation of the mucous membrane of the stomach (gastritis), stomach ulcers, and eventually to cancer of the stomach on the basis of this chronic state of irritation. Here the mucous membrane is so damaged by persistent inflammatory reaction that the production of hydrochloric acid becomes impossible. Its organic point of attack is withdrawn from the astral body. It can no longer fulfil its physiological function which consists in secretion, and retires disinterestedly. Atypical epithelial and glandular growths, which destroy the organ, are the result. The most common seat of stomach carcinoma is in the pyloric region.

It is interesting that even without organic changes taking place, but for purely psychological reasons, the secretion of acid can be temporarily interrupted, e.g. aversion to food. The astral body withdraws and does not concern itself sufficiently with the organs. A long-lasting or complete failure of acid secretion leads to severe damage to the whole digestion, including the formation of blood. It leads also to the familiar pattern of symptoms known as 'essential hypochrome anaemia', an iron-deficiency anaemia, in which the absorption of iron is upset due to the lack of hydrochloric acid. In pernicious anaemia, too, there is an acidity. But here other factors come into it as well.

In curative eurythmy it is important to know *when* to use 'H' or 'Sch', or both sounds together. It is evident from the description of the way in which these two consonants work and from the development of the pathological conditions, that is, as long as the disorders still lie primarily in the emotional region, that we can intervene prophylactically through these sounds with a loosening or activating effect.

Indeed, even damage which has already become organic can be affected. We have to allow ourselves to be guided by the *appearance* and by the gesture in the movements.

If we recall once more the 'H'-gesture, we can understand how a release, a liberation of the astral body which is too firmly embedded in the organs, takes place through it and thereby produces better, more thorough respiration and a strengthening of the etheric–physical complex which is then no longer under pressure from the astral body.

A person's body often indicates stomach trouble. If there is too much acidity present in the stomach, the facial expression is often 'sour' too. One sees very clearly that the organic processes are bound up with the emotional life because of the strong connection between the astral body and illnesses of the stomach, much more so than is the case with other organs. Someone who has a stomach complaint swallows everything down without digesting it sufficiently. He gets all tied up and cannot get free from himself.

At certain periods of life the proper integration of the astral body with the other members of the being takes on a particularly critical form. It is often accompanied by stomach trouble. In a child this crisis period comes shortly after birth, in the pyloric spasms which lead to vomiting and can endanger life itself. Again at puberty, the tendency towards pains in the stomach appears, combined with headaches. These symptoms often begin in the ninth year. The tendency to vomit in the first months of pregnancy is universally known.

The gesture 'Sch' emerges as suitable when the movement of the stomach is diminished. It is also to be preferred to 'H' for vomiting in a pregnant woman, but should only be used here with the greatest caution. (For the use of curative eurythmy during pregnancy see Chapter 3, pp. 19-20.) Experience shows that 'Sch' should be applied a great deal where there is a tendency towards anacidity, while for superacidity 'H' would always be indicated. To summarize, it could perhaps be said: we always think of the 'H'-exercise when the astral body is too firmly anchored in the stomach region and free contraction and expansion cannot take place. On the other hand, 'Sch' is applied when one wants to get the astral body more involved in the processes which take place in the stomach, that is, to intensify the digestive processes, to stimulate the production of acid, and to further the advance of the food pulp in the intestines.

One exercise should be mentioned here which is akin to 'eurythmic laughter', although it has already been fully discussed in the section on the 'A'-sound. It is 'A-Veneration' (pp. 24-5). The 'H'-movement with the shoulders leads us straight into the gesture for reverence. We open out and prepare to receive reverently into ourselves something more sublime. This exercise effects a strengthening of the life forces.

Also in the eurythmical presentation of the marvellous combination of sounds in the word 'Hallelujah' which expresses, 'I purify myself from all that hinders me in beholding the Godhead', 'H' stands at the beginning and the end.

The sounds 'D' and 'T'

In the Curative Eurythmy Course these two sounds represent 'a force which strengthens the activity of the bowels when they are constipated'. Through 'D' and 'T' it is possible to 'counteract many an obstruction'. The physiological effect lies 'in the digestion of the food itself'.

The organism begins to dispose of the food which has been eaten in the mouth or in the stomach, at least as far as carbohydrates and proteins are concerned, and this is continued in the subsequent part of the intestines, the duodenum. All foodstuffs have to lose their own functional forces and structure, so that they may become suitable building-stones for the substance of individual organs. This takes place, as we have already explained elsewhere, through the action of digestive juices and ferments which gradually complete the process of breaking down the food. The process of digestion of fats takes place in the duodenum through the action of the bile and the digestive juices of the pancreas.

In this part of the intestine the conversion of food takes place through the ego-organization until it is almost of an inorganic, mineral nature. It works in the bile and in the ferment of the pancreas. All matter that comes into the realm of the ego-organization has first to be destroyed so that out of this nothingness it can be taken up in the process of building up *human* substance. In the small intestines this activity of the ego-organization takes place in the realm of the etheric. The predominance of the etheric is seen physically in alkalescence.

The acid environment of the stomach indicates the predominant activity of the astral body, as has already been explained in the section on the sounds 'H' and 'Sch'.

The changeover of the digestion from the stomach to the small intestine is especially interesting physiologically. With the peristaltic movements of the stomach the acidified food pulp arrives at the pylorus. This gate-keeper between the stomach and duodenum, however, does not open at each contraction, but only when the acid food pulp already in the duodenum has been neutralized by the alkaline digestive juices. There is, therefore, a pause before the pylorus reopens for the next portion. We see here a physiological difference in the sides between right and left. Left, the acid activity of the stomach is directed mainly by the astral body; right, the activity of the small intestines is going on in an etheric-alkaline medium.

Any remedy to be effective in this area must have the power to hold the balance of this physiological asymmetry between right and left and must assist in the destruction of the food even to the point where it reaches the dead, mineral state; that is, it must strengthen the ego-organization. In curative eurythmy this can be achieved by the sound 'T'.

*

First let us try to bring before ourselves the power of this sound. In the old Mysteries, 'T' was experienced as the power in the holy word 'Tao' which unites one with Nature as created by the Father-Being. '"Tat wam asi" = "This art thou"—sounded forth to man from all creation. In "Tao" the Atlantean felt the essential harmony of the Divine in Nature.' [23 August 1906.] This was perceived not by the intelligence of the head, but by the heart.

The 'T'-gesture in eurythmy can bring us a similar experience today. It is a solemn movement leading from above downwards. 'This "Tao", "T", is really the sound which has to be felt as representing something of the greatest importance. We may even go so far as to say that it contains within it creative forces, forces which also have a radiating, indicating quality, but with "T" it is more especially a radiance which streams from heaven down onto the earth. There is a weightiness about the sound, and at the same time also a radiance. Thus we can say: "T" is the streaming of forces from above downwards.'

In order to show the effectiveness of 'T' we must remind ourselves of some familiar, general anthroposophical facts.

Our heart and blood organization has undergone a process of gradual condensation out of etheric streams. This took place in the evolution of the earth at a time when the physical body was being transformed, so that it could become a suitable dwelling place for an ego-being. The course of the circulation was laid down with the heart as the central organ. Today we live in an epoch when this process of condensation is beginning to dissolve again. The etheric forces, which have been condensed in the first place into organs and systems of organs, must not go beyond a certain point of density. A turning-point has to be reached which leads then to the etheric forces becoming free again from solid substance. But this does not happen in all the organs simultaneously. This turning-back has already begun for the heart, and this is one of the reasons why illnesses of the heart are so common nowadays.

In the lecture-cycle *Wonders of the World, Ordeals of the Soul and Revelations of the Spirit*, Rudolf Steiner describes how the blood 'is diluted again as it were, in the heart', how 'it dissolves into its smallest physical particles and returns again to its etheric form ... The blood reverts to its etheric form, etheric streams are continually passing upwards from the heart to the human head'. We could not perceive anything of the world, but only that which comes up out of our own inner organs, if these etheric streams were not continually flowing upwards from the heart to the head. There they 'wash and spray' around a 'delicate and important organ of the brain', the so-called pineal gland (epiphysis), to which they have a 'direct relationship'. The epiphysis has, together with the pituitary gland (hypophysis), a significant function. In *Occult Physiology* it is stated that 'we have here, at a certain, definite point in the human *physical* organism, the external *physical expression* of the *co-operation of soul and body*'. This is the 'entrance gate from the sense-world to the supersensible'. Therefore, 'the information to be gained from orthodox science with regard to these organs is very inadequate'. Epiphysis and hypophysis lie opposite to one another anatomically, like two poles. Between them we have the third ventricle through which the cerebrospinal fluid flows and which is bounded, besides the pituitary gland and the pineal gland, by highly important parts of the brain (mid-brain, thalamus, hypothalamus). Rudolf Steiner further amplifies his description of the pituitary and pineal glands by saying that there are two etheric currents 'which oppose each other under the greatest possible tension, just as two electric currents oppose each other. If a balance is brought about between these two currents, then a conception has become a memory-picture and has incorporated itself in the ether-body'.

Thus, from the anatomical-physical point of view, this subcortical region is the place where our sense-perceptions and thoughts are transformed into permanent memories through the activity of the pineal and pituitary glands. They are impressed upon our ether-body, and thereby it becomes the bearer of our personality between birth and death. For only when we can connect from day to day what we have learnt and experienced in life do we have a lasting personality–character. It is that part of the brain with the pineal gland of which it was said that it is 'washed and sprayed around' by etheric currents, streaming from the heart to the head.

Let us be quite clear that we are dealing with two streams meeting each other: the first etheric current streaming upwards from the heart to the head and there washing around the middle part of the brain, and a second current in which live the perceptions coming from the sense-world.

We see the 'T'-gesture before us. If we experience, as we look at it, the underlying zodiacal gesture for Leo, the Lion, which radiates glowing enthusiasm, and if we raise our arms with this feeling, then we enhance the etheric stream flowing up from the heart. This encounters the one radiating down from above.

We see these two streams clearly in the eurythmy figure for 'T', the one rising up from the heart, transforming the shape of the head into a vessel, and the other falling slowly from above and being received by this vessel. In doing the curative eurythmy 'T' we should strive to bring out these two aspects as ideally as possible. Only then will the full physiological effect of 'T' be achieved.

*

Today we see many illnesses in which the pathological opposite may be observed of what Rudolf Steiner describes as positive functions of that portion of the brain mentioned above. They are post-encephalitic disorders, which for the most part have their seat in the subcortical zone of the brain, that is, in the area around the third ventricle. From the great number of brain-damaged children which we are able to observe in our curative institutions we will describe those for whom the 'T'-exercise is suitable. They are the children suffering from kinetic restlessness and a definite personality disturbance. They are usually well formed, the body is well proportioned, but they have a vacant and empty look. They are continually fidgeting. The movements are meaningless, unrhythmical and chaotic; it is quite impossible for the children to control the impulsive movements. If one tries to make purposeful movements with them in eurythmy or painting, one encounters the greatest resistance. They are tormented by their organs. In the worst cases they can think of nothing but satisfying hunger and thirst, that is, the organic needs. Many of them are completely shut off from the world of thought and ideas. It is difficult to teach them anything at school, even when the ordinary intelligence is unimpaired. It is not possible for them to take in ideas about the world, and so they cannot make any memory-pictures for themselves either. In a certain sense, the etheric body remains empty; the personality is not formed. 'For people with disturbances of this kind only the present moment exists, as it were; for them there is no past from which they can learn, no future to be considered; altogether a terrible disturbance which destroys the central human functions.' [Hans Asperger, *Heilpaedagogik*, 1952.]

Several curative eurythmists have observed that these children can often be appealed to only through the sound 'T'.

Today, the change in the personality occasioned by this illness is largely attributed to the brain centres and tracts, through whose failure the symptoms of the illness appear, and it is not taken into account that these symptoms are only what is left over from the processes in the higher members. This opinion cannot lead to prophylactic measures. We find a great variety of degrees and modifications at all stages of what appears so final and often seems inaccessible in brain-damaged children, since destruction of the organs has already set in. Yet it is through this knowledge that we are in a position to be able to help.

*

In 'T' we have been introduced to a gesture through which the ego, streaming downwards from above, is greatly strengthened and is impressed into the etheric life.

So far we have been considering this in the realms of head and heart.

Now the effect of the 'T'-sound in the digestive processes can become comprehensible. An X-jump with the legs belongs to the curative eurythmy 'T'-exercise, while with the 'D'-jump the feet carry out a similar movement to that of the arms.

Obstipation, occurring through malfunctioning in these parts, is usually characterized by obstinate constipation and can easily turn to diarrhoea, followed quickly by renewed constipation.

*

The gesture 'D' shows a pointing towards something, radiating towards something. It was the gesture with which the Indian pupil was instructed by his 'Dada' who pointed significantly towards something— drawing attention—setting free. The sound 'D' also comes from the zodiacal sphere of the Lion, and the gesture of 'fiery enthusiasm' belongs to it as well. If the blood process is stimulated by this gesture, then the warmth of the heart flows into the movement and 'D' leads us, permeated by warmth, out into the surrounding world. The gesture, pointing outwards, cannot then become a nervous, restless fluttering. Blood and nerves make a harmonious whole. The physiological processes which are manifested in 'D' and 'T' become comprehensible from the chapter 'Blood and Nerve' in the book *Fundamentals of Therapy*. There the threefold meeting between blood and nerve is described.

Blood, which is permeated by the astral body, and nerve, also permeated by the astral body, work together in the middle system of man. This is apparent in 'D'. Through the nerve-process, the movement, throbbing with the blood, becomes controlled in pointing at external things. Blood and nerve are balanced in 'D'.

The scope of this movement is also applicable in the middle part of man and it has a healing effect in the early stages of nervous illnesses. Many neuroses arise because people find no satisfaction in their profession or in their personal life. The connection with the surrounding world, which is a concern of the heart, is lost. Interest is restricted to what is directly connected with one's own life. A real contact with other people and with the affairs of the soul and spirit in life cannot be found.

We can understand that 'D' and 'T' unfold their activity in all three realms of the threefold man.

What occurs between blood and nerve in the brain becomes visible to us in 'T'. Blood that has been etherealized encounters the ego-permeated nerve-sense activity. In the middle we have 'D' as the balance between blood and nerve. In the metabolic realm both sounds work for a better digestion of foodstuff. Here 'nerves permeated from within mainly by the action of the etheric organism, work with the blood substance that is paramountly subject to the activity of the ego-organization'.

The sounds 'G' and 'K'

In our studies so far we have been looking at the fields of activity of 'H' and 'Sch' in the stomach, of 'D' and 'T' in the duodenum, and of the sounds 'L', 'R', 'S' in the small intestines. Now we come to the sounds 'G', 'K' and 'Q', which work upon the large intestine, upon the evacuation of the bowel.

In the Curative Eurythmy Course Rudolf Steiner states that in the sounds 'G', 'K' and 'Q' (in which the effect of 'Q' corresponds to that of 'K') we have a movement 'which promotes the movement of the intestine itself'. It stimulates 'the progress, the inner mechanism of the intestines, when the intestines themselves stop'.

The words 'inner mechanism' are used here. Mechanism is something that is subject to the laws of the earth. In the colon the digestive activity begins to adapt itself again to the laws of Nature, while the movements we were talking about before come more under purely cosmic influences. This is also shown in the shape taken on by the large intestine. The small intestine is able to move freely and is only fixed at the beginning to the duodenum, and again where it joins the large intestine. Otherwise it twists and coils around in varying positions. On the other hand, the large intestine is fixed in its position. It has ascending, transverse and descending parts. In the parallel formation of the ascending and descending portions we see the adjustment to the forces of gravity which are also working in our limbs. The contents of the large intestine, which at the beginning are still liquid–pulpy, get firmer as they proceed on their way; the liquid is reabsorbed to some extent by the mucous membrane of the walls of the colon. What remains is the sediment and this has to be excreted. Should a disturbance occur in the motility of the large intestine in connection with which spastic and atonic conditions are usually combined, then this excretory process stops. The sediment remains too long in the intestine and through the nature of the mucous membrane of the colon to absorb liquid it becomes too thick and condensed. The prolonged delay and the resulting reabsorption of virus leads to reaction in the rest of the organism which is manifested in headaches, feelings of repugnance, lazy thinking. To promote the movement of the large intestine, 'G' and 'K' are used effectively. When these two sounds are used correctly, as shown by decades of experience, all aperients can be dispensed with, even in the most difficult cases of constipation, and there has seldom been a failure when this exercise has been done energetically and for an extended period.

It is not difficult, in this case, to deduce the effect from the gesture of the sound. The gesture shows a pushing-away, a warding-off of the external. 'G' is started with a strong movement in the shoulders and it travels down through the upper arm, lower arm, hands and fingers. 'G' is an explosive sound, and like all explosive sounds it leads to what is within asserting its true worth. The movement is held for a moment. The figure is taut, the back of the head and the spine are tense. In this gesture we feel the forces of the upper man overcoming the forces of the lower man. For the upper man this means liberation and relief. The words *genug gierigen Geniessens* (enough of greedy enjoyment) also indicate a pushing away of the lower forces. This subduing of the lower forces is even stronger with the 'K'-gesture. In it, Rudolf Steiner says, we have 'a control of matter by the spirit'. The power inherent in 'K' can only be unfolded properly if the movement is really begun and allowed to flow out from the area around the shoulder and the character felt especially in the upper arm. The effect of 'G', as well as of 'K', is diminished if the pushing-away movement does not begin in the upper arm but is only started peripherally with the hands. In curative eurythmy, 'G' is accompanied by a jump with knees together and feet apart (the X-jump), 'K' by a jump which is made 'with legs spread widely apart' while jumping forwards.

With the application of 'G' and 'K' in cases of severe constipation, the possible range of activity of these sounds is, however, not exhausted. Let us stimulate further consideration by quoting Rudolf Steiner's words about 'G' in the Speech Eurythmy Course:

> The sound 'G', when properly formed—'G G'—signifies an inner *self-strengthening* of the soul-forces, a concentration of everything in the human being which in the ordinary way tends to diffuse and spread itself outwards. It is therefore the sound of speech which, so to speak, holds our being together, in so far as the latter is a vessel for natural forces. This is the sound 'G'... The warding-off of everything external and the welding together of everything inward is expressed in the gesture for 'G'.

What does this statement mean? What is it that 'in the ordinary way tends to diffuse and spread itself outwards'? What are the 'natural forces' with which the human being 'allows himself to be filled, as it were'? We are dealing here with a problem that is connected with the etherization of foodstuffs and with the threefold current of substance in the human organism. The natural force which fills us inwardly is the foodstuff which is transformed through the fluid and gaseous states to the condition of warmth-ether and which through the power of the ego is condensed again and as solid substance is secreted and incorporated into the organism. 'Before any substance can reappear in the human organism, it must first have been changed into an entirely volatile etheric warmth form and then changed back again into what appears in living form in the human organism . . .' This warmth-ether has 'a strong disposition to absorb into itself what radiates inwards, what streams inwards, as forces from world-spaces'. 'The warmth-etherized earth-matter' is imbued with these spiritual forces, 'streams then into all man's internal regions, and builds up, in that it resolidifies, the material basis of the several organs of the body . . . With the help of what comes from the spiritual cosmos, it then [the mineral substance which has been transformed into warmth-ether. *Author's note.*] becomes resolidified into the earthly condition.' [10 November 1923.]

An 'excretory process' takes place into the physical realm from out of the warmth-ether realm, into which the foodstuff has been raised. In this way *human* organ-substance is formed. We have here an 'inward excretion'—it could even be called 'in-cretion'.

It is not only the crude physiological elimination taking place in the large intestine which can be upset. It is not only a stoppage in the physical realm that is expressed in the non-functioning of the bowel elimination, that can be removed by means of 'G' and 'K'. If we find that the solid matter in the organism is not sufficiently formed in a patient, that the 'material basis of the several organs' is inadequate, then this is connected with a disturbance in the 'inner excretory process', with a defective 'in-cretion'. With 'G' we can overcome this cessation of the substance-forming stream, and make it flow again. Physical matter is again precipitated out of the etheric. 'To avert all things external and to weld together the inner life' means: to check the destructive forces, to concentrate the inner upbuilding forces. Muscular dystrophy, diseases in the growth of the organs, changes in the shape of the body are indications for the extended scope of these sounds.

'G' and 'K' are also used for defective formation of the teeth. The teeth are the most mineralized part of man. Around the 7th year a child begins to get his second teeth. It can be seen from his appearance that he is now emerging from the childish–watery–rotund state. It is as though he bursts out of the watery element into the solid. This is significant for the whole configuration of the child. In this process the figure gets its shape and the powers of thought are released. If this does not take place properly it can be seen in the malformation of the teeth. Corrective action must then be taken. However, consideration should be given not only to the teeth, but above all the disturbed process of mineralization should be controlled. The pushing forces of 'G' and 'K' help the organism to 'secrete' solid substance conformable to the ego.

We have tried to complete the so-called 'classic' application of 'G' and 'K' for constipation from the characterization of these sounds given in the Speech Eurythmy Course. We hope, thereby, to have aroused interest in this important sound and that people will occupy themselves more with it and not just stick to its effect in the intestinal region. A private remark made by Rudolf Steiner about 'G' can be of some help here: 'G' 'governs with the forces of the higher world, and is served by the forces of the lower world.'

The sounds 'B' and 'P'

If one is looking for an ideal example of the 'B'-gesture, there arises before the mind's eye the wonderful figure of the *Sistine Madonna*. The figure seems to float in the air and yet walks with feet firmly on the clouds. She has conceived one of the angelic babes from on high, and it now rests upon her arm. She has drawn a blue mantle around the Child in loving protection—we see before us the ideal representation of envelopment. The soul-forces of the spirit-child in every human being are enfolded in this way. The Word of God, the true, primeval human being, has been clothed in many a sheath since the beginning of the Saturn evolution. The astral sheath of the soul was evolved on the moon. In it lies the capacity of developing love from its lowest to its highest form. Now the astral sheath, which is so far developed that it is allowed to carry the Infant Jesus, is made manifest to us in the *Sistine Madonna*. Purifying and healing forces for man's sheaths flow from this picture and Rudolf Steiner often gave the advice to let restless children look at the picture of the *Sistine Madonna* before going to sleep, at the same time gently stroking their head.

The protective, enveloping quality of 'B' has always been felt. Many words in our language beginning with 'B' show this business of protecting and enveloping: blade, blossom—the 'B' envelops something which wants to unfold itself in 'L' and express its nature in the vowel sound.

When, in 1924, in the Speech Eurythmy Course, Rudolf Steiner had the gesture for 'B' demonstrated, he emphasized that it was through holding the arms at *different* levels that the enveloping quality of 'B' could be felt. He wanted to have expressed 'that which is *around* something'. He designated 'B' as a 'protecting gesture', in which what is seeking to be protected and the enveloper are both expressed at the same time. As an example he chose a child whom one embraces protectively with both arms. Whenever one makes a 'B'-gesture one should feel that something is being held in the hollow space which is enclosed by the arms.

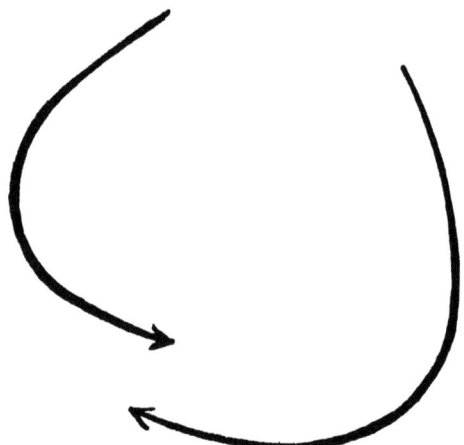

In 'P', the encircling, enveloping gesture of 'B' with its blue veil is changed into large, pointed, forms, coming from the outside inwards, suggesting in flowing movement something that envelops.

In curative eurythmy we use 'B' and 'P' to work on the 'inner digestion', on all the digestive activity going on in the blood vessels, but especially the digestive activity in the kidneys'.

The alimentary canal from the mouth to the anus belongs to the outer world; it is involuted outer world. The separation which takes place there between the substances assimilated from outside and the digestive juices secreted by the human being is only a preparation—the inner digestion begins on the other side of the intestinal wall, in the blood and lymphatic streams. The food which has passed through a zero point is re-enlivened and taken up into one's own ether body. This has already been discussed in the description of the sound 'L'.

It is the kidney system that mediates in the assimilation into the astral body of the re-enlivened foodstuff. The common view held today is that the kidney is solely an organ of excretion. Can we also detect functions of this organ which are of importance for the whole constitution, for the functioning of the whole organism? We need only look at patients with kidney disease. Serious disorders often appear at the surface. The skin becomes flaccid, grey in colour, the eyes are lustreless and consciousness is dulled. We have in the kidneys a radiating organ for the astral body. The astral first builds its physical sheaths from air and light. Then gradually an organ is formed as a physical starting-point. Primarily, therefore, the kidney system is an operative organ for the astral body. It follows from this that, as a secondary function, the kidneys also excrete outwards. From the kidneys the astral body radiates through the whole fluid organization. And thereby the relationship is established between soul-experience and kidney function. Materially, this means that what is assimilated from the metabolism by the kidney system streams out radially into the organism, to the surface of the skin and to the head system. Thus the radiation to the periphery is diminished if the kidneys are diseased. How this radiating stream is rounded off and shaped by the head is described in Chapter 8. In the Curative Eurythmy Course a great deal is said about how these forces, raying out from below and shaping from above, can be influenced, on the one hand by the consonants, and on the other hand by the vowels. Rudolf Steiner's reference to the fact that in performing any consonantal eurythmy the back of the head, lungs, liver and kidneys become luminous, that 'a glittering and sparkling' begins, that a whole 'copy-in-light of the excretory process of the kidneys' becomes visible, applies particularly to the consonant 'B'. The things described here are among those for which the curative eurythmist should try to acquire an eye. This is not easy to do and can only be achieved through continual practice. Direct observation while watching the patient as he does his exercises can reveal more than all the intellectual pondering.

If the astral activity is too weak then the radial streaming upwards of substance from the kidneys is insufficient. There is not enough substance coming to meet the formative head forces. The contact between them and the distribution of matter is inadequate. Metabolism relapses into itself: haemorrhoids, heavy menstruation, deposits of a rheumatic nature are the result.

If the astral activity is too intense, or if the physical–etheric organ of the kidneys brings too much resistance to bear on the astral intervention, then pain is caused in the gastro–intestinal tract. The radiation is so strong that congestion, headaches and migraine conditions occur.

We use 'B' for all the illnesses we have mentioned which are the result of the radiation from the kidneys being either too weak or too strong. When doing the 'B'-exercises we must make sure that the whole back is involved—the movement begins from the back and with a strong gesture is finished off firmly at the front. Since the sounds themselves are our teachers, we can learn and deduce a great deal from the difficulties which the patients have in carrying out the gestures. Some patients find it difficult to perform gestures that condense out of the wide spaces of the spiritual world in order to enwrap themselves in them. Others find it almost impossible to bring this gesture to a proper conclusion as an explosive sound should do. 'B' depends very much on the qualities of firmness and conclusiveness. This is especially obvious when the exercise is given for rheumatism. Rheumatic people can be either fat or thin. Those who tend towards plumpness do the broad, open part of the 'B' very well, but then the gesture gets blurred around the edges. The thin ones, on the other hand, pay very little attention to the beginning of the exercise but go straight into the firm forward movement.

In curative eurythmy we do 'B' with the legs as well. It has to be started gently from the hips. The knees must remain loose and the feet placed lightly and without contortion. This is often an extremely difficult task. Nearly all patients who need 'B' begin with stiff hips, straining knees and uncertain or hard setting-down of the foot. The exercise is only successful when the patient can manage to form the 'B' properly with the legs. The 'B'-exercise is done with arms and legs, both sides together or alternately, getting faster and faster, and it is done for about five minutes at a time.

*

For the treatment of migraine a metamorphosed B-execise is specified with the soul exercises. We form the 'B' and at the same time bend the knees so that we are in a crouching position and quite enveloped by the 'B'. From this position we quickly stretch the whole body, simultaneously letting the 'B' dissolve downwards. When it is done according to these directions, ten times consecutively, and then after a pause another ten times, it is a strenuous but effective exercise. It should only be done during the intervals between migraines, never during an attack. Before the start of an attack the patient often complains of urine retention. As the migraine passes off a urinary flood can occur. From this we see how strong the connection is between this illness and the activity of the kidneys.

'B' and 'P' work especially on the excretion of water by the kidneys. Experience has taught that both sounds have a strong effect on any kind of water retention. The 'P'-gesture, with its decisive movement from outside inwards and from above downwards, has an even stronger effect on the excretory function than 'B'. Neither should one hesitate to do the 'P'-exercise even with patients who have dropsy very badly. It cannot be done then with a jump—this is seldom possible anyway—but it can be done standing, alternatively with the right and left leg, and a great deal can be achieved with it.

Like all consonants 'B' also greatly assists the breathing-in process. Its healing effect is seen in the great craving for air often felt by kidney sufferers, and in the difficulty they experience in their breathing.

*

In the therapeutic use of the sounds 'B' and 'P' we can always bear in mind that they directly affect the astral body. The activity of the astral body, spreading out from the kidney system, is still firmly fixed in the organic—bound to the world of the desires and passions. Nervous anxiety and disturbed conditions of various kinds have their cause here. In such cases the 'B'-gesture, done very calmly and quietly, purifies and cleanses the astral body. It is, therefore, understandable that 'B' and 'P' occur in the sound sequence for the emotionally disturbed: 'M-N-B-P-A-U'.

For many patients who come to their curative eurythmy straight from the rush of daily life, it is good to do the 'B' as a preparation for the other exercises. This enveloping gesture brings the desired tranquillity which is essential for the success of curative eurythmy. The 'B'-exercise is particularly important for children living in large cities and exposed in such high degree to the detrimental influences of civilization. Frequently these children also lack the security which the mother and the family should give. With 'B' one can try to compensate, at least in part, for this predisposition to damage due to exposure.

And so we have to come back again to the picture with which we started: the cosmic ideal of the Virgin who lays the protective wrap around the Child in her arms. As the sounds 'B' and 'P' work from out of this cosmic archetypal image of the Virgin and bring their powers to bear on human beings, so there are cosmic archetypal images underlying all the other sound gestures, out of which they are born (see Chapter 10).

The one who is giving the curative eurythmy should renew in himself again and again this picture-world, giving strength to the sounds from within—from whence flow the healing forces in which the patient can submerge himself even if he knows nothing of what we have just been saying.

The sound 'M'

Even in the gesture, 'M' shows its physiological effectiveness. Both arms and hands move towards each other. The one arm is geared more to the stream of formative forces coming from above, the other to the stream of growth forces working from below. They are harmoniously united in the middle by the 'M'. Mean, meso- (in composition), middle—the words show how 'M' expresses the balancing forces of the middle. The polarities of the organs of the digestive-limb system and those of the nerve-sense system find their equilibrium in the rhythmic system. The digestive processes are continued in the rhythm of the blood, the head forces in the breathing process. The balance between blood and breath is achieved. Inhalation comes under the influence of the metabolism, while the head forces dominate in exhalation. Thus in the rhythmic system we have the metabolic-limb pole predominating in the breathing-in, alternating with the predominance of the nerve pole in the breathing-out.

In general the consonants have their effect on inhalation through the digestion. In this, 'M' is an exception in that it has more influence on exhalation.

This is made visible in the way the body is held when making the 'M'-gesture. The upper part of the body leans somewhat forward and has a slight preponderance over the lower part of the body. The relation between lower and upper is stressed by the character shown in the small of the back, as it is represented in the eurythmy figure. If one looks at this posture, or does it oneself, one experiences directly a strengthening of the breathing-out. One does not *think* about breathing-out, but one takes up the position of 'M' and breathing-out follows.

In maintaining the balance between these polarities and bringing harmony to the middle region of man, 'M' creates the 'human being whose forces are held in balance'.

The human being as such becomes visible in his archetypal etheric form. 'M' works from out of the zodiacal sign of Aquarius, the Water-bearer. The name 'Waterman' is the old designation for the etheric man, as it was once thought of within the Creation. Adjusting the flow of juices from below upwards, from above downwards, controlling destruction and restoration, these are the living, weaving tasks of the etheric body. We can assist this with 'M'. It has been found in working with patients that the meeting of the upper and lower arm movement often lies outside the body and does not go out from the middle properly. This latter can always be achieved if special care is taken with the participation of the upper arm. It is necessary that the adjustment shall take place wholly *within* the human being.

In the harmony of one's own being, 'M' can bring about an intelligent comprehension of the surrounding world through the exhaled breath. It leads to a deeper involvement in things, a union with them, and thus to an understanding of them. 'M' is that which 'comprehends everything, which is carried over into the breath so that it conforms to everything and understands everything'.

Thus the therapeutic side of 'M' also becomes understandable. It works 'as a regulator on the whole metabolic organism, the limb organism'. 'Especially if it is done during the development period, it adjusts the sexual urges.'

If 'M' is used at the time of puberty, it is done with the peewit-step which is performed in the following way: one leg is placed before the other. In hopping forwards the back leg hits the front leg at the back of the knee and in so doing the front leg is flung slightly upwards. The peewit-step is practised first with one leg in front and then the other. It is more difficult to do the same movement hopping backwards. It can be still further intensified by doing it forwards and backwards alternately. This complicated, flinging leg movement is accompanied by making an 'M' with the arms very calmly and quietly.

This exercise has been drawn from what actually happens physically at puberty. Puberty causes great changes to take place in the human organism. The reproductive glands begin to work, the thymus gland of childhood diminishes, the entire endocrinal control apparatus undergoes a transposition, new hormones appear in the secretory flow. The digestive system gains superiority, the voice becomes deeper owing to increased metabolism. The limb movements become more conscious and consequently awkwardness and embarrassment frequently occur at this age. The human being is now mature, he attains creative forces, generative powers. To begin with, these irritate him, they trouble him— a new harmony, a new balance must be found. In the educational field we try to guide these newly awakened faculties towards an understanding of the world. For the human being is really only completely of this world at puberty. His own inner being can now face the external world more independently, and he has to come to terms with it in all its aspects and in his dealings with it.

All this takes place in the organic subconsciousness and breaks through confusedly into the emotional realm. The whole organism can be thrown into disorder if the processes of digestion and the sexual urges become too intrusive. 'M' assists all that is aimed at in the educational field at this critical period of life. It has a harmonizing effect and with its controlled gesture brings the still tumultous, newly awakened forces into the breathing-out process. Thus they can prove themselves in the right way by enabling human beings to experience the world around them and other people.

The upward movement of the digestive forces becomes visible to us in the curative eurythmy exercise of the peewit-step with the legs. It demands tremendous control of the movement impulses to perform the quietly breathing 'M' at the same time as the peewit-step. When these two movements are carried out so that they coincide properly, then the digestion, rising up from below, is calmed down by the 'M' from the middle.

*

The sound 'M' is known to us from the ancient Indian culture in the syllable 'AUM'. Rudolf Steiner says about it that this syllable finishes with 'M' because 'particularly through this sound the whole human being is regulated by his digestive-limb organism'. It was practised in order to train the human being physically, to strengthen him in his will, but at the same time to help him to learn restraint, self-control, and to be able to keep hold of himself.

In this exercise the child is allowed to become aware of his own proficiency. The remarks made in the Curative Eurythmy Course may be recalled: 'In that moment when the child says as he breathes out: there now, I am really a very fine chap; when he experiences his breathing-out in such a way that he seems to himself to be a fine fellow, as if he felt his powers, as if he wanted to impart his powers to the world in breathing-out, when he feels all this, he also feels the corresponding movement of the abdomen, of the limbs, the carriage of the head, in the right way'.

As already mentioned, we perceive 'M' in the compensating activity of the various etheric streams. The weaving of the etheric becomes most clear to us in the plant. The sap flowing upwards from the region of the roots encounters the shaping forces active in light and warmth. In the middle part of the plant, in the leaf, they are in harmony with each other. The plant blossoms when the forces of light and warmth working in the air prevail, growth is repressed and an astralization of the etheric plant-formation begins.

In the human being, too, there is an etheric, plant-like process. A plant does not, however, grow in him; everything remains functional and procedural. The important point is that the direction of this process is exactly the opposite to that of plant growth. The plant sinks its roots into the earth and grows upwards towards the flowering process. In man, the plant nature is rooted in the head and grows downwards to what is flower-like. This flowering process, the astralization, is to be found in the region of the kidneys and the sexual organs. And this astralization process begins with puberty.

This reversal of the plant process in the human being is very significant in the use of plants for nutritional and therapeutic purposes. It is only mentioned here in order to deepen our understanding of the 'M' sound.

What is clear and lucid outside in Nature is involved, and therefore complicated, in the human being.

In childhood the growth forces coming from above downwards are linked with the ego activity which works from the head and warms the organism through and through. The reversal takes place gradually between the change of teeth and puberty and reaches its culmination in the ninth to tenth year. The warming process, going out from the head, diminishes and would become weaker and weaker if the ego did not begin to enter into and become part of the stream flowing from below upwards, begin to be co-ordinated into the digestive process, into the blood process and the circulation as far as the breath. The ego activity must now take over the warming process from below upwards. The crisis which the child goes through around 9-10 years of age is largely caused by this process of readjustment. The ego, working now from below, meets with the upper stream and must be balanced in the middle part of man in the breathing and blood process. In this period of life the breath and the blood adopt the ratio of 1:4 which is to remain for life. For a healthy life much depends upon this process taking place properly. If this harmonization in the middle region is achieved, then the young person, as he grows up, can find his connection with the world around him. The forces of his environment become effective for him—the bodily constitution is changed, the chest broadens out. The true middle of the human being, with its own surrounding world, is born. In the practice of curative eurythmy it is almost daily borne in upon us how many predispositions to illness arise when the extremes of head and will are enormously developed while the middle part of man is stunted.

Thus, 'M' is the sound that is used against the troublesome urges of sexuality—it creates harmony in the middle between the upper and lower being of man, it leads to an understanding of the world around. It is therefore suitable for making puberty into a truly real process of earthly maturity.

*

A further exercise which restores a balance is 'M with head shaking'. The 'M'-movement is accompanied by a movement of the head from side to side. This head movement is performed faster and faster—which is not easy in conjunction with the calm movement of the arms in 'M'. 'By means of a detour through the etheric body' this exercise has a soothing effect on 'irregularities in the abdomen'. This exercise may be done while seated in a relaxed position. In special cases it has been prescribed in certain rhythms, e.g. exercise three days consecutively, then four days break or even six days break. But in any case it should only be done when there is no pain. Very often the patients who require this exercise feel the need themselves, when they have period pains, to move the head to and fro to loosen the muscles as they feel the cramp goes out from the head and neck.

The balance between the upper and lower forces is also upset in this indisposition. The 'M with peewit-step' works against the troublesome sexual processes. The 'M with head shaking' restores harmony when the nerve-sense pole works too strongly on the lower processes. Physiologically, the stream working from above downwards must predominate so that the period, which is an eliminatory process, can enter. If this process, directed downwards from above, becomes *too* strong, then the processes of the lower body, which should proceed unconsciously in the organic sphere, become too conscious—pain is the result and menstrual irregularity. From the picture of the plant turned upside down in man it follows that the root process, working out from the head, overcomes the flowering fruiting process during the period. Biologically it is known that during the period women do not have a good influence on flowers, that flowers in their vicinity tend to wilt. Rudolf Steiner, too, points out that this piece of folklore is founded on fact. [18 April 1921.]

Through the head shaking that accompanies the 'M' in this exercise, we are able to soften the dominating forces of the head and through the 'M' to establish equilibrium again.

As a harmonizing factor 'M' is a good remedy for insomnia. It is given in many sequence-exercises (see Chapters 11–12). It is discussed there, too, as an exercise for the breathing and asthma.

'M' is appropriate whenever we wish to help the human being in his efforts to achieve and maintain his human state of balance. In this respect Rudolf Steiner's explanation of the relationship of the sounds 'A–M' and 'H–M' are specially impressive. The strength of 'S' 'as the actual ahrimanic sound' is reduced by the 'M'. 'Its ahrimanic strength' is taken from it by the 'M'. On the other hand, 'H' is connected with the luciferic, and can lead to arrogance. If 'H' is allowed 'to go slowly over into an "M"' then 'the sting is taken' from the luciferic element. 'This movement is really as if we would hold Lucifer back.' 'M' stands like a balancing power in the middle between the 'H'-sound, aspiring to the luciferic, and the 'S'-sound directed towards the ahrimanic side. The sculptured wooden Group at the Goetheanum springs to mind: the Representative of Humanity between Ahriman and Lucifer. In 'M' we have at our disposal a power which enables us to modify the forces of temptation coming from two sides by strengthening our own middle region. It is that power which today is in danger of being lost—through which alone we can preserve our humanity.

The sound 'N'

Among the consonants 'N' is, to a certain extent, unique in the way it works. Nearly all the consonants affect intestinal activity when there is a tendency to severe constipation; 'N' is the only one we use for diarrhoea.

Acute diarrhoea can be caused by a number of things; infection, bad food, upset stomach. This does not mean that curative eurythmy has to be used immediately. Relief will be sought through appropriate dietetic measures, medicaments and applications of warmth. It is recognized that people of an unstable disposition can get diarrhoea from excitement, shock, fear, stage-fright.

If a person tends to get diarrhoea with emotional excitement there is often a constitutional weakness in the lower being. The vegetative or autonomic nervous systems, which as the name implies is connected with the life-processes which are independent of the will, is in such people 'unstable' and easily swayed by outside influences. Emotion, shock, continual worry, can all lead to far-reaching injuries in this sphere. In such cases, where soul-experiences are too strong and affect even the physical activity of the intestines, we add to 'N' the exercise of the sound 'U'. Through its power to overcome fear and straighten the limbs 'U' works right into the bowel organization.

If the tendency to diarrhoea becomes constitutional it has usually to do with the sense-nerve process, which is most concentrated in the head and at the circumference of the skin of the human being, getting pushed too far into the inner being and breaking through into the digestion. What ought to be working in the consciousness pole of man, in the thinking process, becomes displaced and interposes itself into the digestive processes. The result can be serious diarrhoea, even typhoid conditions.

How are we to get from this an idea of how 'N' works? In the 'N'-gesture we move the hands, the fingertips, towards something—this can even be the air—touch it lightly and draw the movement back again. We make only a fleeting connection with something and quickly draw back again. In the whole body, especially the head, something is holding back. The back of the head is emphasized. Fingers and toes have been permeated with sensitive touch by the soul-and-spirit. In this gesture there is only a slender connection with the surrounding world which is regarded with detachment. Let us remind ourselves of the 'M'-gesture in which one is united in loving sympathy with things, feels at one with them and so understands them. The understanding is different in the 'N'-gesture. We touch the phenomena of the external world and withdraw again in order to be able to understand them objectively. We could almost call this a negation of awareness, something taking place with antipathy. The perceptive power of the middle system, of the heart, is working in 'M'; in 'N' it is that of the head. Without these powers we could never form a clear concept. This becomes clear when we observe retarded, mentally defective children in their development; they can often stand somewhere for a long time, given up to their surroundings, entirely drawn out into the surrounding world of Nature. But they do not really take it in, they cannot detach themselves from it nor form any thoughts about it. Thus it is difficult for them to come to any intellectual realization of the world. For just such a child Rudolf Steiner gave the sequence 'R-L-M-N' and commented: 'In "N" there is that which brings one back to a rational way of thought'. [*Curative Education.*]

'N' can be used to help children to be better able to form concepts, to further the intellectual understanding. It has a favourable effect on children who—in their feeling, be it stressed—attach themselves sympathetically, usually in a happy frame of mind, to people and things, but whose thinking powers are developed only with difficulty.

Sympathy and antipathy are the fundamental polarities of our soul-life. We have seen that 'M' strengthens the forces of sympathy, and the forces of antipathy are made stronger through 'N'. These forces of antipathy are just as necessary in the organic life as in the life of the soul. The forces of the head, which we use mentally in the formation of thoughts, organically lead to the formation of nerves and bones, to the formation of hard substance. The hardest bone is at the back of the head. The effect produced by 'N' has also an important starting-point there. We know the poor development of the back part of the head in cases where the bone-forming tendencies are too weak, e.g. in rickety children, and to a great extent in Down's syndrome children. In the latter all inclination to form abstract thoughts is absent. They give themselves up to life in pure sympathy; their bones remain soft for a long time. As well as other exercises 'U' and 'N' strengthen the formative forces which are lacking in them. When the development of the back of the head is defective it is even possible to stimulate the plastic forces through 'N'.

From the sentence quoted above, 'In "N" there is that which brings one back to a rational way of thought,' it is possible to understand its effect on diarrhoea. For, as already described, the point is to free the nerve-sense process from the digestion and direct it back to the head organization where it rightly belongs.

*

'N' can also have an effect on the teething process. We shall not now go into the connection between tooth decay and thought processes, the development of either good intelligence or slow-wittedness. It is just mentioned in order to stimulate one's own observation. Just as 'N' is able to form and strengthen the bones at the back of the head which have remained too soft, so too it can counteract softening of the teeth and can be used prophylactically against tooth decay. From the educational field we know that we can influence the process of dentition by training the hands and feet to be skilful and supple, so that the soul is made to go right into the fingers. 'The 'N'-gesture is of great assistance in bringing this about.

I was very impressed some years ago when doing 'N' in a case of acromegaly, an illness in which the extremities of the organism, the tips of the nose, chin, fingers and toes, become coarse and enlarged. They are no longer 'tips' but rather clump-like deformed enlargements. 'N', with its accent on the sensitive, properly formed toes and fingertips, was the obvious choice as treatment and it had good effect.

Such experiences make one realize how important it is for penetration right to the periphery to be really achieved at the beginning of the 'N' exercise. Only then is the drawing-back of the second phase of the movement effective. 'N' leads us to a calm control of our organism and allows it, even physically, to become the basis of our consciousness.

The sound 'F'

How Rudolf Steiner spoke about 'F' in the lectures in the summer of 1924 (*Eurythmy as Visible Speech*) will remain unforgettable to all those who were present. One marvelled to hear that in the ancient Mysteries a sound was regarded as having such comprehensive reality. Among other things he said: 'In uttering the sound "F" one felt that the wisdom contained in the Word became conscious.' He indicated that 'F' could only be rightly understood when one is able to comprehend, even now, what is expressed in a little known formula of the Egyptian Mysteries: '*If thou wouldst proclaim the nature of Isis who knows the past, the present and the future and from whom the veil can never entirely be lifted, then thou must do this in the sound "F"*.' 'To fill oneself with the being of Isis in the process of breathing, to experience Isis in the out-going breath-stream, is what lies within the sound "F".' [25 June 1924.]

The experience of wisdom in the breathing process was practised in 'F' at that time. 'Know, that I know', is what one wanted to say with 'F'. It is difficult to experience 'F' 'in an age when the conception of language is so impoverished'. This can be a certain consolation to us, if at first we have difficulty in grasping the sublimity of such a sound.

Only a few indications were given in the Curative Eurythmy Course for 'F' and at first they are not easy to understand. 'Then we have the sound "F", "V". Here we are dealing with something psychic ... We have here a movement which should be practised when it is found *that the discharge of urine is not in order*. If, for any reason, it is necessary to stimulate this, then this movement should be done.'

If one has worked for a long time with 'F', the inner content of these words is revealed and becomes a guide for the application of the sound.

'F' is used with great success for bed-wetting children. Now bed-wetting is one of the important symptoms of childish, hysterical derangement and by observing the composition of this malady we can learn much about the efficacy of the sound 'F' as it is described in the Curative Education Course.

The basis of childish, hysterical derangement is a constitutionally too weak connection between the etheric and physical bodies in the abdominal organs. In every organ it is necessary to have a particular relationship in the co-operation of the higher members of the being—just as hydrogen and oxygen will only form water in the ratio of 2:1 (H_2O). In the abdominal organs the physical body and etheric body have to be closely united with one another. When this is not the case, as in childish hysteria, widespread disorders can occur. The organs become too pervious and therefore the ego and astral body do not find sufficient support in them; they go through the surface of the organ and flow away. While in epilepsy the ego and astral body are obstructed because of resistance at the surface of the organs, in hysteria the organs are like sieves. Ego and astral body trickle out and not enough astral and ego activity remains behind in the organs. This leakage is to be taken literally—the secretions, particularly perspiration and micturition, are affected by it.

Rudolf Steiner points out that bedwetting in children will only be seen 'in its proper perspective' when it is considered in this light. 'Whenever you have a case of bed-wetting, you can assume that the astral body is running out. Every kind of secretion and excretion has to do with the activity of the astral body and the ego-organization. These must be in order if the secretions and excretions are to be normal.'

Let us now consider the psychic disturbances that occur with this kind of illness. Because of the constitutional anomalies of the organs, the ego and astral body get through into the surrounding world, intensively but uncontrolled. With an instinctive feeling for the events happening around one, a half subconscious knowledge arises. Too strong an attachment to the world around leads, in its turn, to hypersensitivity and thereby to too strong a withdrawal into oneself. Instability in the life of the soul develops which vacillates between flowing out and shrinking back into itself.

In many bed-wetters the symptoms of hysteria are only slight; nor is the cause always to be found in these constitutional irregularities. Bed-wetting is, as we know, a widespread affliction. It is often to be found in children who grow up in difficult outer circumstances, e.g. a broken marriage. The continual effects of shock to which the children are exposed without protection can lead to a certain loosening between the etheric and the physical body, through which corresponding symptoms then appear.

Here are some examples of actual case histories.

A boy was conspicuous in that he had wide-open eyes and also very large ears. His senses were wide open and he was very much at the mercy of his sense-impressions. He lived only on the surface of things, with curiosity and without really grasping the impressions and absorbing them into his life of soul. This boy was a very bad bet-wetter.

There is another type of child: fair, delicate, excitable, oversensitive. With every excitement, whether from joy or from shock, they have trouble in preventing the bladder function coming into action. The weakness of the bladder is usually seen less in the wetting by night than by day. The astral body here also lives too much in the periphery. This instability, again, is caused by constitutional hysteria.

In some children bed-wetting takes place only at crises in their development, for instance at puberty when with the discharge of urine self-pollution (semen ejection) can occur.

*

Let us now turn to the sound-gesture for 'F' in order to learn from it its application in curative eurythmy.

In the year 1912 Rudolf Steiner spoke about the 'F'-gesture, saying that it should be seen as the reaction to a challenging, external influence—as reaction to an exciting, challenging external world. In a picture, he made it clear what the 'F'-gesture expresses. And one is deeply moved by this picture which Frau Lori Maier-Smits describes in her memoirs somewhat in the following words:

> A man is working in the fields towards evening. The small birds are perched quietly in the unmoving tree-tops, singing their evening song. A tranquil little stream, murmuring gently, winds through the meadows. The golden light of evening lies over the deep and peaceful landscape. Suddenly a violent gust of wind bends and shakes the tree-tops. The birds fly off in alarm—the stream is whipped up—racing clouds chase across the sun . . . and the man responds to this agitation in the world around him with the 'F'-gesture.

Life in the human being is stirred by agitation in the life of Nature around him. The Greek experienced this agitated life of the outer world as the same as that within himself. The etheric life forces outside him awakened etheric life forces in his organs and created thoughts in him. Our individual etheric body is connected with the universal world ether; there was a time in our pre-earthly life when we drew our individual ether body from the universal world-ether. And it is this world-wisdom, lying hidden within us, which responds to the stirrings of the external world through the stimulus of the 'F'-gesture.

When it was said in 1924, ' "F" is wisdom in exhalation', then this is a somewhat different aspect of the same occurrence: wisdom within responds to wisdom without. The physical-organically active wisdom in us answers the wisdom working outside in Nature. Thus through 'F' an image is presented of Persephone, who descends to the underworld (i.e. into our physical body) and enters into a dialogue with her mother Demeter who is the wisdom of Nature, working in all that is growing and dying in the plant world.

The ego and astral body enter into the wisdom of the etheric body through 'F' and experience it in exhalation. It is clear that this is not possible when the ego and astral body have nothing to hold them in the organs and drain away, as was described for the symptomatic picture of hysteria.

We can achieve two things through the controlled guidance of the curative eurythmy 'F'-exercise. Etheric body and physical body which are too loosely interwoven are pulled more firmly together. The 'F'-jump is particularly important here. One jumps from the toes, falls back onto the heels, jumps again from the toes, falls back again onto the heels, and so on. In this way a rhythm is set up which is just what we want for the lower organization. Emotionally disturbed children who are bed-wetters can often not do this jump without help. One can assist the child by taking hold of both ankles and pressing them down firmly but gently onto the floor after each jump. With this emphatic movement of the feet we press the etheric body more firmly into the physical organization in the lower part of man's being. Consequently the astral body finds a hold in the consolidated organs. The aimless, painful, subconscious reaction to the outer world disappears. Now the child can respond in his breathing to the challenge of the world. The etheric–watery element is no longer poured out in excessive secretion and the powers of the etheric body can become fruitful in the understanding of the world around.

The power of 'F' must be felt in every moment of the movement. The posture must not collapse—not even when one gets back onto the heels. In all cases of bed-wetting the 'F'-gesture is directed downwards.

Since children with a hysterical constitution are often very unprotected, it is good to combine the 'F'-exercise with the sound 'B'. When the bed-wetting occurs at puberty, then the appropriate combination would be 'M'.

Besides the hysterical set of symptoms, there are other psychopathic conditions which are obviously connected with changes in the secretion of perspiration and urine. In certain cases it will be necessary to seek medical advice as to what extent the 'F' should be used along with other exercises.

CHAPTER 10

Consonantal and Zodiacal Forces in the Human Form

Even in 1920, before the Curative Eurythmy Course had been given, Rudolf Steiner said in the course for doctors: 'And if one begins to study how differently vowel eurythmy, for instance, works in the lower part of man and in the upper part, and again, the consonantal, formative eurythmy works in the lower and in the upper part of man, then it can be seen that in eurythmy one can also look for an important therapeutic element.' [6 April 1920.]

So far we have considered the consonants as they affect the lower part of the human being, how they almost all influence the digestive activity and bring this rather chaotic activity into the rhythm of circulation and breathing, and how some of them work right into the inner structure of the head.

Now there is still another side to the effect produced by the consonants. That is the one which goes out from the head, forming and shaping the human form. In the Curative Eurythmy Course our attention is directed towards forces which play around the head. They are forces which 'create a kind of aura about us'. The consonantal forces are meant here which unfold their plasticity around and through the head-organization. 'Thus we have first and foremost the moulding work in the head-organization and in this way we shall be able to stimulate such a head-organization which, to some extent, has been left behind. So if we are dealing with someone who is feeble-minded, with someone in whom we can confirm that also physically his head-organization is not in order, then we get him to do consonantal eurythmy.'

Rudolf Steiner nearly always prescribed consonants in curative eurythmy for cases of paralysis and deformation. We have to ask ourselves how we are to understand the effect of the consonants working from the head on the human figure. More detailed explanations are to be found in the following lectures:

Die Gestaltung des Menschen als Ergebnis kosmischer Wirkungen (not translated).

Man in the Light of Occultism, Theosophy and Philosophy.
Eurythmy as Visible Speech.

This brings us to the cosmic aspect of the consonantal forces at home in the twelvefoldness of the zodiac. The physical human figure has been created out of these forces of the zodiac into a twelvefold unity as follows:

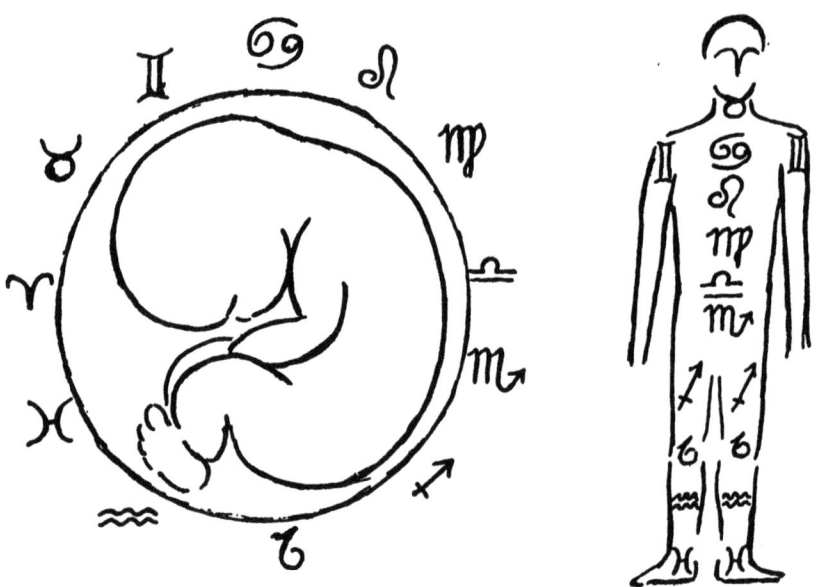

Aries—Head
Taurus—Throat and larynx
Gemini—Symmetral plane
Cancer—Chest
Leo—Heart
Virgo—Solar plexus

Libra—Hips
Scorpio—Reproductive organs
Sagittarius—Thighs
Capricorn—Knees
Aquarius—Shins
Pisces—Feet

This affinity of the human figure with the 12 constellations of the zodiac has been known since olden times and is to be found in many a medieval book. But we can only gain an understanding of them and learn to use them for curative eurythmy therapy from the knowledge imparted by Rudolf Steiner of the zodiacal gestures and the explanatory notes which he gave to go with them.

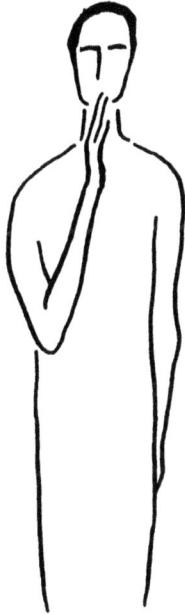

Aries—'V'—'The Event'

From the constellation of Aries formative forces stream forth to act upon the roundness of the human head. The form of the head is a complete image of the universe. The spherically formed head is separated off from the cosmos as a spherical image at birth—that is the 'Event'.

In old pictures the Ram is usually looking backwards. And 'this backward look of the Ram represents the backward look of man to the universe that lives within him'. Man finds the relationship to his own human form in this backward look to the universe.

If a child is born with deformities of the head, or it cannot attain an upright position, then we try to stimulate the plastic forces of the head with the consonant 'V'. Thus, if we are dealing with deformities of the body, we use consonants. However, if we want to affect the inner power of the ego to stand upright, then vowels, e.g. 'A' and 'U', are the appropriate exercises.

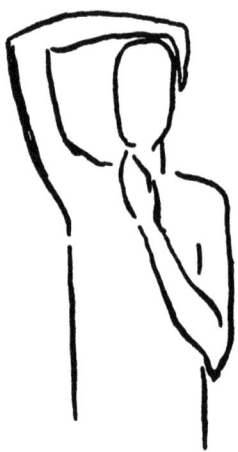

Taurus—'R'—'Will, Deed'

In Aries man is looking back towards the cosmos. Now those forces are beginning to stir which lead him to action, to reply to the cosmos. The larynx, and the organs connected with it, are created out of the constellation of Taurus, the Bull, and human speech is born out of inner activity. The entire human form is directed towards vocal expression, in sound and speech. Once again deformities in this realm can be removed by practising the sound 'R'.

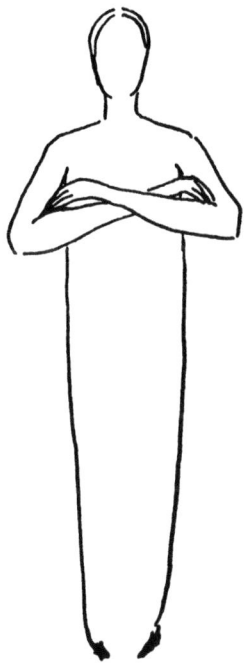

Gemini—'H'—'Capacity for Will'

In the constellation Gemini the human being now receives his bilateral, symmetrical arrangement. The Twins are basically the right and the left side in the human being which merge with one another on the plane of symmetry. Man thereby becomes 'Capable of Will', that is, he can touch himself, he can take hold of himself, and that gives him the capacity for 'doing'. What could we accomplish on earth if we had not two legs and two arms! This plane of symmetry extends even to the two hemispheres of the brain.

With children who do not know their own bodily form and, therefore, do not perform an act of will, we let them practise taking hold of their right ear with the left hand, or touching their left little toe with the right forefinger, and so on, so that in this way they may become aware of themselves.

Moreover, the inner taking-hold of oneself by the ego is connected with the vowel sound 'E'—but the body is able to do this through establishing the plane of symmetry under the influence of the zodiacal sign of Gemini.

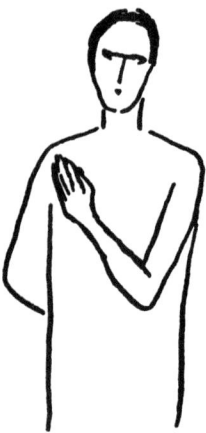

Cancer—'F'—'Initiative'

The formation of the body continues to go from the outside to the inside. The gesture for Gemini leads us from the outside world as far as our skin where we feel ourselves. In Cancer, however, we begin to detach ourselves from the cosmic surroundings. The gesture presents an encircling of the breast from left to right, from front to back. This gesture divides the inner from the outer and encloses it. The chest cavity is formed which encloses our heart and lungs, as protection for our inner world. Thus, 'Initiative', or 'Impulse to Action' can be aroused within us.

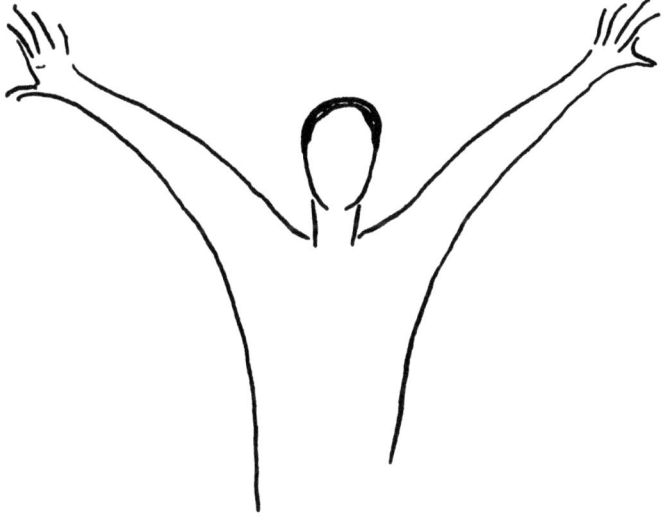

Leo—'D', 'T'—'Fiery Enthusiasm'

We now come to that which makes us inwardly complete, wherein the very kernel of our being lies. Heart and circulation originate here; they pervade the whole human being, occupy us from the centre to the periphery—blood vessels go everywhere, the blood flows everywhere. The actual physical-bodily organ of the heart and the blood vessels belongs absolutely to the human configuration as a product of the twelvefoldness of the zodiac. 'If we compare the limbs, for instance, which we have already considered, with the circulation of the blood, there we have something which takes place completely within us, something that is entirely enclosed.' We have now got to the constellation of the Lion, an animal with a well-developed heart. The gesture for Leo leads us from the nucleus of the heart in 'Fiery Enthusiasm' out into space, there to be made fruitful in 'T' or 'D'.

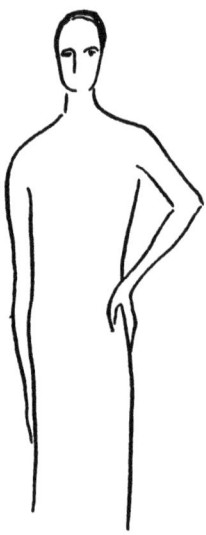

Virgo—'B', 'P'—'Rational Sobriety'

In the creation of the human form we have now reached the innermost being, the heart. However, communication with the outer world still exists through the lungs.

In the realm of the creative forces of Virgo we find an inner organic region which is no longer open to the outside world: spleen, liver, gall-bladder, etc. and the 'brain' which belongs to them, the solar plexus. 'We have here a part of the human form which we could call the actual core of our being, the core in a bodily connection—and it is of significance that it is without connection to the outer world.' In this region of the body which is formed by the constellation of Virgo, the soul of man can attain maturity in the peace of seclusion. The Virgin is depicted with an ear of corn which is the symbol of maturity. 'Rational Sobriety', the zodiacal gesture of Virgo, follows the fiery enthusiasm with which the gesture of Leo is turned towards the cosmos. The soothing effect of the sounds 'B' and 'P' on the whole region of the solar plexus has already been described.

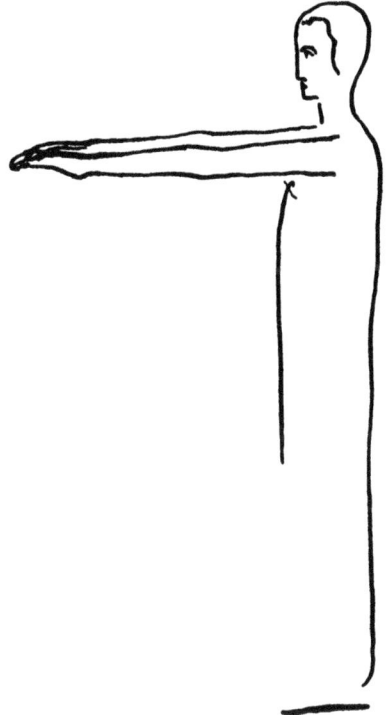

Libra—'Ts'—'Weighing up the Premises of Thought'

Having taken hold of the inner being, the gesture for Libra leads us now to seek a balance between the inner and the outer. In this region the hips are formed, where we find the balance for our deportment. The human being begins to integrate himself from out of his own inner being, through his limbs into the earthly forces. The gesture, consisting of outstretched arms and hands laid one on top of the other, is difficult to achieve without a balanced posture. It is a gesture which only a human being can make as he stands upright in an easy balance, and who alone is capable of freely 'Weighing up Thought'.

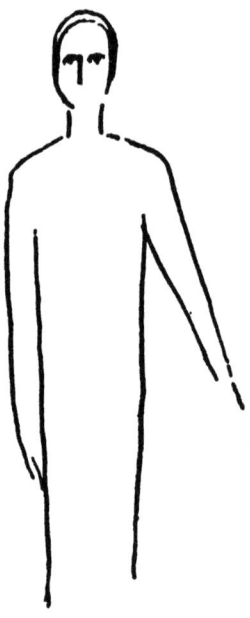

Scorpio—'S', 'Z'—'The Understanding'

In the Scales we try to find the integration with the outer world. In Scorpio we receive the outer world into ourselves, through the food we eat as well as through sense perception. But everything that enters into us from the outer world is, in a certain way, poison—'a kind of venomous sting'. We have to come to terms with it and resist it. In resisting what comes from outside, the inner organism is shaped. In the lower part of man the digestive and sexual organs are created—in the head, the frontal brain, with which we form thoughts about our perceptions.

This constellation of the zodiac is represented by the Scorpion with its poisonous sting, as well as by the Eagle which portrays the powers of thought.

Consonantal and Zodiacal Forces in the Human Form 143

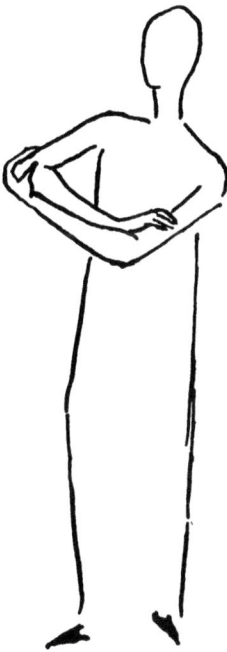

Sagittarius—'G', 'K'—'The Resolve'

The gesture for Sagittarius shows the special emphasis laid on the upper arms and thighs. The forming activity goes more and more from the inside to the outside—from the 'thought' (Scorpio) to the 'Resolve'. Expressed organically this means: the limbs are formed which are adapted to the laws of the earth.

This movement, followed up with a 'G', can be used successfully in curative eurythmy for people who get abdominal pains.

144   *Fundamental Principles of Curative Eurythmy*

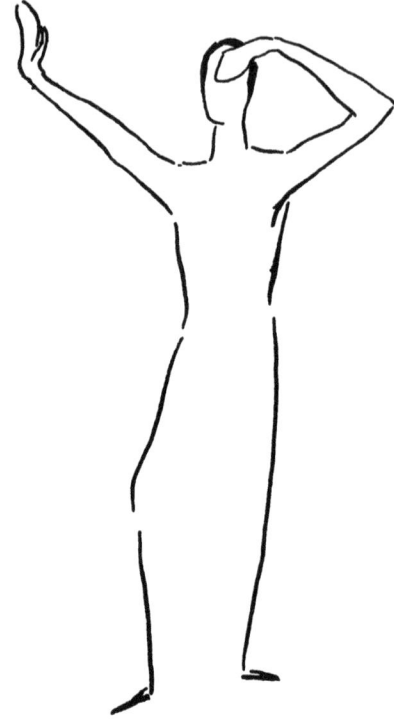

Capricorn—'L'—'The Bringing of Thought into Relationship with the World'

Out of this region comes the formation of the knee in the human body. Anatomically the knee is of great interest. It is very dramatic in its formation. The crossed ligaments and the knee-cap, which does not belong to any group of bones, give great freedom of movement. The balance of movement has to be found in the knee between the forces of gravity, rising upwards from the feet and the lower legs, and the formative forces of the upper leg coming from within. So the knee appears to us as having been formed out of a whirlpool of currents.

And there is especially a lot of free etheric force around the knee—as there is round every joint to a certain extent. This was well-known to the people of bygone centuries; some pictures and sculptures by old masters show vigorous, whirling movements in the flow of the garments around the knees. Goethe, too, indicates this when Dr Marianus speaks about the Mater Gloriosa in *Faust*, Part II.

Um sie verschlingen	Light clouds are circling
Sich leichte Wölkchen,	Around her splendour,—
Sind Büsserinnen,	Penitent women
Ein zartes Völkchen,	Of natures tender,
Um Ihre Knie	Her *knees* embracing
Den Aether *schlürfend,*	*Ether* respiring,
Gnade bedürfend.	Mercy requiring.

(Bayard Taylor's translation.)

In the gesture for Capricorn there is an area of great tension between the left hand, which touches the forehead, and the right hand, which is stretched out in front. It is here that 'L' endeavours to come into existence—in the 'Bringing of Thought into Relationship with the World' that sound comes to birth which, as can be seen, holding itself within itself, overcomes gravity.

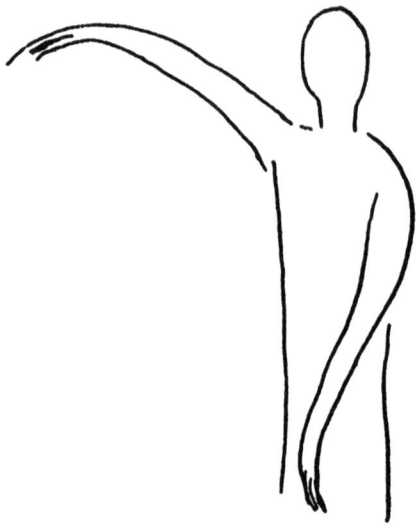

Aquarius—'M'—'The Human Being in a State of Balance'

The lower leg and the forearm are formed by the influence of the forces of Aquarius. The Aquarius gesture shows the balancing flow of movement in the swinging up and down, down and up, of the arms.

If we look at the two bones of the forearm we see that the joint between upper and lower arm, the elbow, is formed entirely by the ulna which narrows as it passes downwards to the wrist, ending in a slight expansion to form the head of the ulna. The radius begins with a broad head at the wrist, tapering upwards towards the elbow. The up–down, down–up flow is clearly seen in these two bones. The same goes for the lower leg, although for reasons of stability both joints are carried by the powerful shin bones, while the fibula has become a subsidiary bone.

Consonantal and Zodiacal Forces in the Human Form   147

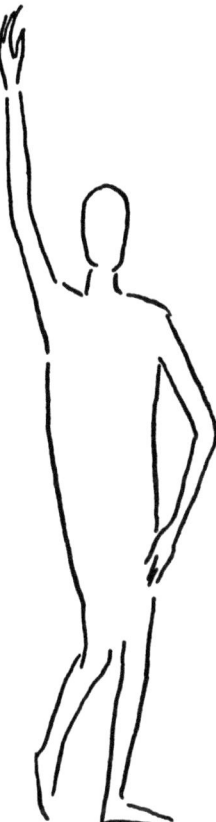

Pisces—'N'—'The Event has become Destiny'

The feet form themselves under the influence of the constellation of Pisces. The body of the human being is now complete. It stands there in freedom between the higher and lower forces—the feet adapted to tread the earth, and yet, as the gesture of the Fishes shows, ready to rise again. By means of the feet man is able to move over the earth, seeking his destiny.

The feet have great flexibility and are perfectly adapted to the earth. There is the firm, strong heel—the toes, sensitively feeling out the way we tread—the ball, which enables the foot to roll smoothly at every step, and finally the wonderful arch of the instep which gives elasticity to the rise and fall of each step. The threefoldness of the human frame is seen once more in the foot.

The zodiacal forces, forming and shaping the body, are described from three points of view.

The lectures given in the year 1912 start from the spiritual being of man—the 'I'. We are looking for an external, physically perceptible expression of the ego. This is the human form. And so we recognize how in its construction the human form is so fashioned that an ego can unfold therein as a spiritual being, adapted to earthly conditions and endowed with an upright posture and the gift of speech. See the table below:

1 Aries — Uprightness
2 Taurus — Beginnings of sound formation
3 Gemini — Symmetry
4 Cancer — Seclusion
5 Leo — Enclosing of what is within
6 Virgo — Physical separation from the outer world
7 Libra — Balance
8 Scorpio — Reproductive organs
9 Sagittarius — Thigh
10 Capricorn — Knees
11 Aquarius — Lower leg
12 Pisces — Feet

The twelvefold figure of man can also be divided into groups of three times seven, as follows:

Upper Man	*Middle Man*	*Lower Man*
♈ Upright position	♊ Head and feet	♓ Feet
♉ Forward direction	♋ Enveloping of chest	♒ Lower leg
♊ Symmetry	♌ Inner, heart	♑ Knees
♐ Upper arm	♍ Innermost processes are active	♐ Thigh
♑ Elbow	♎ Balance	♏ Reproductive organs
♒ Forearm	♏ Reproductive organs	♎ Balance
♓ Hands	♐ Thigh	♍ Kidneys, solar plexus

(In this table the signs of the zodiac have been used instead of the names of constellations.)

This arrangement gives us the important therapeutic indication that we have to apply the same consonantal and zodiacal gestures for the upper arm, elbow, forearm and hands as for the thighs, knees, lower legs and feet.

In the 1921 lectures the human form is presented as it originates from the inner activity of the movements of the constellations of the zodiac. A certain threefoldness underlies this arrangement: the first four signs of the zodiac work on the human form from outside, from the universe; the next four form the inner man; and the last four work from within outwards, forming the limbs with which the four original vocations of man are connected.

It could be tabulated as follows:

1 Aries — Uprightness
2 Taurus — Looking to the universe and absorbing the mobility of the universe
3 Gemini — Taking hold of oneself (touching)
4 Cancer — Enfolding oneself
5 Leo — The filling-out-from-within
6 Virgo — Ripening
7 Libra — Finding the way into the inorganic world; seeking the balance
8 Scorpio — The poisonous sting
9 Sagittarius — Huntsman
10 Capricorn — Animal husbandman
11 Aquarius — Arable husbandman
12 Pisces — Tradesman

*

In the year 1924 Rudolf Steiner gave indications for yet another way of understanding the working of the zodiac from the aspect of the three soul activities, beginning with feeling:

Feeling in relationship to the Lion
Thinking to the Scorpion
Willing to the Bull
Harmonizing of thinking, feeling and willing to the Waterman

*

We use the zodiacal gestures for deformities of the body and paralysis. Whether we use these 'forms which arise out of the human being' directly, in such cases, or only the consonants arising out of the gestures, depends on the situation. In general, we are extremely cautious about using the zodiacal gestures in curative eurythmy. It can be quite sufficient for these cosmic movements to be alive within the curative eurythmist.

The question is often asked, whether the consonants should be done differently according to whether they are supposed to work on the digestive system or on the plastic forces emanating from the head. First of all let it be said that the whole etheric organism always does the sound as well, even if the movement is carried out by the little finger only.

Nevertheless, the exercises do change according to whether attention has been directed towards the effect of the consonants on the digestion or on the form. For the digestion we perform the consonants together with their specific jumps—either singly or in sequences as required. For variations in the bodily structure, deformities, postural defects, paralysis, etc. the 12 kinds of formative forces of the constellation give us guidance, especially as regards the actual region of the body. Even in cases of severe paralysis, the capacity for movement can be reawakened if the consonant is done over the corresponding region of the body, e.g. 'M' over the lower leg or forearm, 'L' over the knee, and so forth. It is often possible to stimulate movement in the fingers or toes by doing the 'N' with one's own hands on the fingers or toes of the patient.

If we want to work on the digestion we appeal to the consonantal forces in the elements—in solid matter, in the watery, in the airy and in the warmth elements.

If we want to work on the actual form, we call more upon the cosmic forces of the consonants.

CHAPTER 11

Consonant Sequences

In the following chapter the consonant sequences which Rudolf Steiner prescribed for certain illnesses are combined in groups.

We may regard them as study material to which we can always return to work out a course of treatment in an individual case.

In sequence exercises one sound always runs directly into the next one. Occasionally the separate sounds are practised by themselves.

'L-M'

This is one of the most used consonant sequences. 'L' strengthens the breathing-in, while 'M' carries us over to the breathing-out. Hence we have a breathing exercise built up from sound. And here it depends very much on the way in which they are done. 'L' must be done strongly, making full use of the joint of the shoulder and upper arm, so that one goes directly over into the 'M' and thus into the breathing-out.

All one's effort in curative eurythmy should be directed towards the breathing process. We do not do any breathing exercises which have been consciously thought out, such as are employed in many methods of remedial gymnastics, but we see to it that in every curative eurythmy exercise the breathing is harmonious and deep. The change in the breathing can be directly experienced and put to use. If calm, deep breathing is achieved with the exercise, it is good then to prolong it for a little while consciously, but only as long as the breathing remains undisturbed.

'L-M-S-U'

This exercise was given in the Curative Education Course which stimulates the activity of the etheric body and points in the same direction. (See also Chapter 9 under 'S'.)

'L–M–S'

For Basedow's disease [goitre]. In this illness the astral body tends to become stiff, to follow its own inclinations and avoids the regulating and restraining power of the ego-organization. In the trembling movements, the protruding eyes, the uncontrollable anxiety and increasing exhaustion, we see the physical manifestations of the dislocation of the higher members of the being.

A patient with goitre, who was herself a curative eurythmist, set herself the exercise of carrying out consciously, for a short time each day, all habitual movements: getting up, going to the door, opening it, and so on, always completely concentrated on each particular movement. This helped very much in her recovery.

Long before there was any curative eurythmy, Rudolf Steiner had given the advice to a goitre patient to walk on his heels several times a day.

This same sequence of sounds is also indicated for inflammation of the middle ear (otitis media). The point is that around the ear, but also in the organism as a whole, the etheric body develops too much activity. The breathing activity, but especially the breathing-out, has to be stimulated. This is brought about through 'L–M'. 'S' adds formative forces to the exercise. 'L–M' may be practised with the whole body, and then followed up with smaller 'S' movements near the ear.

'L–M–N–R'

An exercise prescribed for a patient who suffered from severe psychic depressions, conditions of fear and insomnia. Besides this there were changes in the knees and pains radiating from the neck into the arms and legs.

A patient with inhibitions and depressions during the menses was given the exercise: 'Stiffen your legs and bring your ego in.'

'D–T–L'

Prescribed for a 39-year-old patient who had suffered for 14 years from noticeable tiredness and an increasing need for sleep. The tiredness started in the morning already and grew worse if he did not eat for some time. His stool was irregular, alternating between constipation and diarrhoea. He liked to be alone and also suffered from depression.

'D-T-S'

This was practised with a 35-year-old patient who, since the commencement of menstruation at 11, had been depressive, and since her 18th year had suffered increasingly from pressure on the stomach, eructation, apathy, insomnia and extreme fatigue.

'L-R-T'

This was practised for some time in the Clinic in Arlesheim with a patient who suffered from severe constipation, stomach pressure and nausea. When Rudolf Steiner saw her he confirmed this treatment and added 'M' to these sounds.

'R-S-L'

For obesity. The sequence may be combined with the 'O'-exercise.

'L-M-S-R'

Prescribed for a 17-year-old patient who was exceedingly intellectual and suffered from extreme thinness (anorexia mentalis). Menstruation commenced at the age of 12 years. Two years later, after great strain, the periods ceased again and after every meal she had stomachache which eventually led to a complete refusal of food. In her conduct the patient was over-intellectual and obstinate. Besides other treatment she got this consonant sequence from Rudolf Steiner which her sister who had a similar constitution also had to practise.

'Consonants'

Prescribed for a 26-year-old patient after an attack of manic excitement. He also suffered from insomnia.

'Doing consonants in the imagination' was advised for a patient with hysterical paralysis. She was primarily handicapped in walking.

'Consonants with the feet' were prescribed by Rudolf Steiner for a 50-year-old patient at the beginning of the menopause with an anxiety complex. The periods were irregular and very heavy. Besides which she had had a liver complaint for 20 years.

'Doing consonants'. 'If the formative forces are inadequate, that is to say, the formative activity is unchecked. That is to say, the formative forces, working centrifugally, make the head big, with the result that the imaginative forces cannot penetrate it in the right way.'

'Doing consonants' for a boy of 12¾ years of small stature, intelligent, but tiring quickly mentally, who had worms. Here, too, the imaginative forces are inadequate; the formative forces of the organs are out of control.

'Doing consonants' for deformation of the joints—a lack of imaginative forces.

'Consonants with the head' for a woman patient with climacteric difficulties (especially hot flushes) 'to cool the head'. Additionally, 'M-with-head-shaking', three days consecutively, then miss out six days.

'R–S–L–M'

This was prescribed for a 44-year-old patient who had a bad haemorrhage after a fall, 'because the astral body did not enter properly into the abdominal organs'.

'M–L–R'

For habitual miscarriages. This exercise should only be done by stepping gently or seated.

'L–S–N–R'

This exercise was given to a 40-year-old patient who had suffered for two years from early morning diarrhoea which had started with acute fever. Rudolf Steiner said: 'It all depends on getting iron into the blood, then the conditions will improve. It is indeed almost too late to do this.' We are dealing with putrid disintegration of the blood which provides the breeding ground for parasitic growth. This was the result of ego weakness in the soul organism. 'She lives really as if she were only sitting *on* her body with her ego, and lives astrally.' It was for this reason that she had to do a *lot* of eurythmy—the consonant sequence as directed, especially with the legs, but also with the arms. The exercise was given thus in the Clinic, Arlesheim.

Sometimes other sounds for this case have been mentioned erroneously, e.g. 'L–M–S–R'. But 'N' is particularly important for counteracting diarrhoea.

'R-L-M-N'

Prescribed for a retarded, microcephalous boy who came to the Clinic when be was 9. He had a narrow head, though the lower half of his face was strongly formed. His mouth was always open. His hands and feet were very large and clumsy compared with his body. He liked to talk to his right forefinger as if it were a person which he called 'Bebe Assey'. Rudolf Steiner explained that this was an elemental being which had manifested itself there. Soon after he had started curative eurythmy, the game with 'Bebe Assey' disappeared because he penetrated his hands more fully. When practising the prescribed sequence of consonants more emphasis should be given to the leg movement than to the arms. The aim here should be to stimulate the limbs through the sounds, to benefit the formation of the head and to awaken the intellectual powers. One begins by stimulating the inner movement through 'R', then the organism is made pliant through 'L' which at the same time stimulates inhalation, leading over through 'M' to the process of exhalation, and so directing the awakened powers towards the intellect with 'N'.

'S-R-L-M'

For epilepsy. In contrast to the more usual vowel exercises prescribed for epilepsy, an 18-year-old patient who had only had epileptic fits since her 16th year and often made unco-ordinated, convulsive movements, was given this consonant sequence. In addition it was said: 'indeed, everything which helps the ego-organization.'

*

Some illnesses will be described here in more detail which had to do with handicapped movement and for which Rudolf Steiner gave exercises.

First of all the rheumatic complaints.

'R-L-M'

For chronic muscular rheumatism. A 55-year-old patient, tall and lean, had a great deal of pain in all her muscles. Rudolf Steiner pointed out that too much crystallization had occurred in the wrong places and needles of crystal were deposited throughout the muscular organism, impeding movement and making it very painful. He prescribed that she should make herself into a circle by sitting down and touching her toes with her hands. From this position she should stand up and quickly, do three 'R's (big, curative eurythmy 'R'), then sit again, making the circle, and quickly stand up and do 'L' three times (with X-jump), make the circle again for the third time, stand up and do an 'M' three times (with peewit-step).

This exercise is done in various ways, e.g. as 'O-L-O-R-O-M-O'. So far it has not been possible to discover whether this is another direct suggestion from Rudolf Steiner, or whether it is a variation on the exercise given originally in the Clinic in Arlesheim. It should be remembered, however, that this is an exercise given for *muscular* rheumatism.

It is a different matter when we are dealing with rheumatic illnesses of the joints. Here we have to consider various forms. Acute arthritic rheumatism is seldom treated with curative eurythmy. It is different with chronic illnesses of the joints, where we have to distinguish between inflammatory and degenerative forms.

We can set to work at an early stage on chronic, inflammatory polyarthritis which usually begins slowly. As a preliminary symptom there is often a painful stiffness in all the small joints of the fingers and hands, and frequently, on waking up, there is a furry feeling, as if the hands were wrapped in cotton-wool. Generally the symptoms occur symmetrically in both hands. This can be helped with simple exercises like clenching and unclenching the fists, doing 'L' with all the fingers, doing vowels with all the fingers—especially 'I' and 'O'.

Gradually the primary, inflammatory forms turn into degenerative stages and are then similar to the purely degenerative stiffnesses, to arthroses. These used to be defined as arthritis deformans. Since this word is misleading and implies inflammatory processes, the name was altered. The cartilage which covers the heads of the bones and the intervertebral discs slowly changes; the joints become deformed due to the shrinking and the thickening of the capsule, and finally the bones themselves are also affected. Movements can only be carried out with extreme pain. It is mostly the large joints which are attacked: knees, hips, the small of the back and shoulder joints.

The rheumatic illnesses take place notably between the astral bodies and etheric body which, in the joints, have to be always in a particular reciprocal interplay. If the astral body penetrates too far, then disease in the joints can set in; if this happens where the etheric body is weak, then deformative kinds of disease can easily occur.

In most cases of arthroses there is already a constitutional weakness of the etheric body and frequently the way has been paved for the illness long beforehand by mental strain. Deep-seated sorrow, worry and shock result in the astral body encroaching too far and are the cause of arthroses later on. Rudolf Steiner mentions also in educational courses that the causes of subsequent rheumatism may be found in the early school years.

With inflammatory deformations it will be a matter of doing vowels, especially 'O', to form new cartilage, and 'U' when there are defects in the bones. But the vowel exercises must always be prepared for with consonants when organic deformations are already there. We get exercises such as 'L-R-S-O' or 'L-O','R-O','S-O'.

In arthrosis it depends on the localization. If it begins in the knees, then we do lots of 'L'; if the symptoms are in the neck region with cramped neck muscles and pain radiating into the arms and the back of the head, then we select the exercise 'L-M-N-R' referred to above (see p. 152).

Rudolf Steiner also gave the following exercise for rheumatism in the shoulder region: 'L' with the shoulders only to begin with, then one after the other with the upper arm, forearm, hand and fingers as well, and finally with the shaking 'L'-movement—'shaking out the rheumatism'.

*

Muscular atrophy is another illness which leads to severe restriction of movement. Rudolf Steiner gave the following suggestions.

'P-T-L-R'

For progressive muscular dystrophy, in which the muscles themselves are attacked by a degenerative process. In this patient we were dealing with a juvenile form of the illness which had made its appearance in his 18th year. In his son the illness began when he was only 2 years old. The muscles of the seat and upper thighs on both sides were badly affected. When he was 29 he came to us for treatment. Besides intensive medical therapy and baths, some very complicated curative eurythmy exercises were also prescribed.

1 The consonant sequence 'P–T–L–R'.
2 Five minutes walking in which he should awaken in himself the feeling: 'In my heart there is a root. From it are growing two stems into both my legs making them firm and strong.'

By means of this exercise (1 and 2) the legs soon began to feel very much stronger, so that he could go for two to three hour walks. Rudolf Steiner was very pleased with this progress and gave him the following exercises to do as well:

3 Stand for one and a half minutes on the right leg. At the same time bend the left knee up and think: 'The strength of my whole body is in my left leg.' Then do the same thing for one and a half minutes with the other leg: 'The strength of my whole body is in my right leg.' (It should be specially noted that the strength should flow into the bent-up leg, not into the one that is being stood on!) Then one and a half minutes standing on both legs which are bent slightly at the knees and thinking: 'The strength of my head is in both my legs.' Then repeating the same position for one and a half minutes while thinking: 'The strength of my heart is in both my legs.'

Of course this exercise is not for general use, but it reveals much of the nature of the illness. At first, in the walking exercise, the flow of blood is sent from the heart into the legs. Then the strength of the whole body, the strength of the head and the strength of the heart is sent into the legs. In this disease blood and nerves are not working together properly in the middle region. (For further study see Chapter IV in *Fundamentals of Therapy*.)

In this illness we have to distinguish between various types of muscular atrophy. The disease can come from the central nervous system of the spinal cord—it is then called progressive spinal muscular atrophy. But it can also have its seat at the periphery, in the muscles themselves—then it is called dystrophia muscularis progressiva—or— peripherally in the nerves also—then it is called neurotic progressive muscular atrophy. From these various designations it can be seen that there is no clear definition for this illness.

'**R** three times, **M** once, **B** once' was given to a 30-year-old patient who had been suffering for ten years from muscular atrophy. He had had a fall in childhood. Rudolf Steiner attributed the condition to this injury and said 'that the muscles tend to tear themselves loose and cut off their nourishment'.

In this case Rudolf Steiner began by getting a specimen of his writing; this revealed that the patient could scarcely manage to write the letters '**R**', '**M**' and '**B**', and therefore they were prescribed for him as a curative eurythmy exercise. Rudolf Steiner gave, as well, the instructions only to begin each movement and then to stop—that is, the movement should

This illness can also develop after encephalitis epidemica (sleeping sickness).

'L-A-M-H'

A 32-year-old patient suffered from severe insomnia, lassitude, fatigue and apathy after an attack of influenza in the head three years previously. There was rapid improvement under the medical treatment prescribed by Rudolf Steiner. Energy and joy of life were reawakened.

'L-A-M-H' was practised with her in curative eurythmy. In all similar cases it would be permissible to use the sounds 'L-A' (done especially walking backwards), 'M', to restimulate flexibility, and 'H', which could also be done as eurythmic laughter or as 'A-Veneration'. It is also important to do exercises in which the movement is arrested or which alternate in direction, forwards and backwards, etc. Since walking and standing are difficult we also have to consider 'U' and 'I'. There are many other exercises which can be used in addition, above all 'Rhythms', 'I-A-O', 'Hallelujah'—especially prolonged and consistent practice of curative eurythmy is necessary.

We can look back to a number of such cases among patients in whom the illness could be arrested in its early stages through energetic and continuous practice of curative eurythmy.

*

In three cases of infantile paralysis Rudolf Steiner prescribed curative eurythmy exercises. For further study on the origin and development of poliomyelitis one should refer to the lecture given to the workmen at the Goetheanum on 31 October 1923 and to Dr (med.) Wilhelm zur Linden's explanations in his book: *Infantile Paralysis – Its Recognition and Treatment* (New Knowledge Books, 1958).

'S-R-T'

A 24-year-old patient who had had poliomyelitis when she was 15 was given this exercise to do with her hands. At the beginning paralysis had attacked both legs, bladder and rectum, but was already considerably less severe when, after nine years, she came for treatment. There was still a weakness in both legs and bad lordosis when she stood. A motion of the bowels was only possible with the aid of aperients. Curative eurythmy, combined with medical treatment, was successfully carried on for an extended period of time so that eventually she was able to walk again without hindrance.

'Consonants with the rod'

A little girl of 8 years fell ill with poliomyelitis. Paralysis began in the right leg; the next day the left leg, bladder and intestines were affected. When Rudolf Steiner saw her a year later paralysis of the bladder and intestines was gone, the left leg was much improved, the right leg less so. There was, besides, an inward squint at times. Rudolf Steiner wished to make this last symptom the starting-point for treatment. The exercise consisted of ascertaining first of all the normal focus of vision, and then placing objects about three centimetres beyond this point so that she had to exert herself to see them. Sending all her strength into her eyes, she should say to herself: 'My eye is me.' Moreover she should do 'I' with her feet and say to herself: 'My foot is me.' Later, when she could walk with a stick, she should say to herself: 'My foot is me.' But she should not look down at her feet. All the consonants should be done with a rod, whereby the movement is consciously directed into the paralysed limb.

'L–R–T–P'

This exercise was for a 17-year-old patient who, two years previously, had had a feverish illness with violent headaches. A lumbar puncture had been made because meningitis was suspected, after which all the extremities and the back became paralysed. When the treatment started the paralysis had partially subsided. The muscles of the back and shoulders and the left leg were still badly atrophied, the right leg and upper arms less so; forearms and hands were all right. Rudolf Steiner did not regard this illness as typical infantile paralysis. He blamed the acute chill in the first place, followed by the lumbar puncture for the paralysis. Besides curative eurythmy the patient received intensive medical and embrocational treatment. He liked doing the exercises and made good progress.

The above are three exercises which give important indications, but which also show how each case must be considered afresh in order to adapt the exercises according to the illness. If we are dealing with one-sided paralysis, co-ordinated exercises have to be used as well (see 'I').

In this illness, which people today dread and which Rudolf Steiner also described as 'a wicked evil', we have to ask ourselves whether preventive treatment in movement is possible—whether it would not be possible to recognize gradually which children are susceptible to poliomyelitis. It is known that it is an illness caused by too much hygiene in the cultural complex of our civilized countries.

In his book, Dr zur Linden refers to the assertions made by the anthropologist W. Scheidt who maintains that the illness is more prevalent among left-handed and ambidextrous people in whom the physiological asymmetric development of the body is protracted. This can serve as a hint for the prophylactic measures to be taken, and such a remark makes our efforts to overcome left-handedness seem even more worthwhile.

From Rudolf Steiner we have the indication that in poliomyelitis the cerebellum is paralysed due to lethargy in the back part of the astral body. This would prompt us to strengthen the astral body in the cerebellum through movements. We know that dexterity and orientation in space, the co-ordination of movements, are connected with the cerebellum. Therefore lots of exercises which promote dexterity must be done. Such exercises are: being able to stand on either the heels or the toes; difficult running exercises; writing with a pencil held between the toes; 'Dexterity-E'. The hopping games that children used to play are also very suitable. Nowadays a child, unfortunately, has little opportunity of participating in games which make him skilful in movement—so this, too, has to be learnt anew.

CHAPTER 12

Consonants and Vowels in Mixed Sequences

'L-A', 'L-O'

The simplest mixed sequences are 'L-A' and 'L-O'. These exercises help the cutting of teeth, 'L-A' for the upper jaw, 'L-O' for the lower. 'When we repeat the "L"-movement, for example, several times, we simply have the digestive principle in man thrown upwards into the nerve-senses principle, if the "L"-movement is done in association with an "A"-form.' In this way harmony is created between the digestive principle and the nerve-senses principle in man. The disharmony between upper and lower is clearly shown by malformations of the jaw, or when the teeth grow in the wrong positions, and these exercises may be applied to great advantage as experience among school-children has shown. Even when corrective measures are undertaken, these exercises are important and are designed to transform the constitutional disharmony.

'S-M-A', 'L-M-I', 'T-M-U'

For spastic, one-sided paralysis.

In the book *Fundamentals of Therapy*, as a fourth example, a child with spastic hemiplegia is described who received treatment when he was 4 and 5½ years old. This child was paralysed in the right arm and right leg. The prescribed sequence of sounds shows in the most beautiful way how consonants and vowels can be combined. The transition from consonant to vowel is, in each case, brought about through the 'M' and thereby made easier. 'M', which already guides the organism towards exhalation, stands as a mediator between the power of the consonants in inhalation and that of the vowels in exhalation. This exercise is like a model from which we can learn a great deal.

'S-U', 'L-A'

For chondrodystrophic stunted growth.

The 7½-year old boy had, as always with typical dwarfish growth, particularly short upper arms and a large head; he had a pedantic nature. Besides medicinal therapy he was given the above sequence of sounds which were to be done especially with the feet.

For 'rockers'

Left arm: 'I' — right arm: 'I'
Left arm: 'S' — right arm: 'S'
Left arm: 'R' — right arm: 'R'

This exercise was prescribed for the 6-year-old brother of the previous boy who had been making rocking movements with his upper body during sleep since his fourth year.

This is a widespread complaint which is specially open to the benefits of curative eurythmy. These rocking movements appear in many abnormal children, either forwards and backwards, or from side to side. It can even go so far that the children look for a quiet corner in the daytime too, to make themselves a nest and, humming contentedly, they will rock for hours if they are left alone. It is as if they wanted to return to an embryonic state.

Even in normal children these rocking movements are not uncommon. Indeed, it is often the above-average, gifted children with an unstable nervous system who engage in them.

The exercise itself looks like rocking, especially when the sounds are done alternately, getting faster and faster. Rudolf Steiner made the remark: 'He should really rock, until he sweats.'

'G–K–A–I'

This exercise for stammering has already been mentioned (see Chapter 5, p. 53).

In another case of stammering in a 5-year-old boy who was retarded in his development and who also suffered from head-shaking and bed-wetting, he was told to do lots of eurythmy and curative eurythmy, especially exercises with dumb-bells. These exercises with dumb-bells have the same object in view as those given for epileptic children to practise balancing (see Chapter 4, 'E').

'L–U–O–K–M'

This was given to a boy with kinetic restlessness and fidgetiness. It is not easy for these children, having activated all their forces in 'L' to contract themselves into 'U'. Now they have to form from within the 'O' with which they release their forces from the organism, use them with 'K' to gain control of the limbs and finish harmoniously with 'M'. This exercise can be given in conjunction with 'Fidget-iambus'.

'R–L–S–I'

For feeble-mindedness. [30 June 1924.]

In the Curative Education Course the weak-minded children are described from the point of view of movement. They have the greatest difficulty in translating thought into movement. If they are told, 'Go to the door!' they understand very well, but do not move. With 'R' we begin to activate the astral body, with 'L' the etheric body, with 'S' we bring warmth into the physical body, and finally, the whole being is moved from within through the vowel 'I'.

'M–N–B–P–A–U'

For maniacal children. [30 June 1924.]

In contrast to what was described above, what strikes one here is the great mobility of these children. Arms and legs never wait for a command; they are in perpetual motion anyway. The children want to touch everything without forming an inner connection with things. They often develop certain skills and capabilities; however, once acquired they continue to use them in a stereotyped manner. When they are drawing, for example, they repeat the same profile every time; the same figure appears again and again when they are modelling. They are not creative in any way. We are dealing here with an etheric body that has become stiff; it has acquired certain faculties, but can then only repeat the same thing over and over again. The kinetic disturbance can work itself up to a frenzy. In the exercise sequence we find the sounds 'B' and 'P', which have a soothing effect on these children, forming a protection. 'M' and 'N' work more on loosening the stiffness in the etheric body which can then be affected from within by the polarity of 'A–U'.

These maniacal symptoms should not be confused with a manic condition of excitement. The most striking feature of maniacal illness is the rigidity of the etheric body—in mania the etheric body is loose and offers a basis for unchecked flights of fancy and ideas, for incoherent thinking. For manic conditions of excitement let it be stressed once more that all consonants should be practised, but especially 'F' (see Chapter 11).

The feeble-minded and insane clearly show their illness in the way they move. We can even work in a corrective way on the first tendencies which are still within the limits of normality through movement exercises in eurythmy.

'I-L-M'

For dread of open places (agoraphobia).

Rudolf Steiner said about a patient who suffered from a fear of open places that he produced too much carbon dioxide. With the breathing exercise 'L-M' we deepen the breathing and effect thereby a strong exhalation of carbon dioxide. Calm, regular breathing dispels fear. The effect of 'I' on agoraphobia has already been described (see Chapter 4, 'I'). Rudolf Steiner recommended the patient to dwell on the thought every morning and evening: 'As little as the moon is likely to fall onto the earth, as little need I be afraid.'

'I-O-A—L-M-S'

This was prescribed for a 28-year-old woman who was in a state of fear. After radical changes in her way of life and emigrating to another country, she suffered attacks of dizziness with head noises, paroxysms of weeping, outbreaks of perspiration and phobic conditions. This occurred particularly when she was in a crowd of people. Even as a child she had been afraid at night. Besides which she complained of heavy, painful legs—she had very bad flat feet—palpitations of the heart, and headaches. As well as medical treatment, legs and abdomen were bandaged and during this time the sound sequence was practised with the legs, otherwise it was done with arm movements.

By means of bandages the consciousness is intensified in that particular part of the body and the effect of the curative eurythmy is thereby strengthened.

This patient enjoyed doing the 'I'-exercise very much and sometimes wished that she could always feel as she felt while doing the exercise. When she woke up in the morning in a completely negative mood, it was as if she were transformed, after doing the 'I'-exercise, into a mood of confidence.

'I-A-U—with the legs, L-M-R—with the arms'

This was for a 26-year-old epileptic girl who also suffered from a bad digestion. Attacks occurred at the time of her irregular periods. It was possible to regulate the periods through the application of shoulder straps crossed over at the back and treating the soles of the feet with copper ointment. For her bad digestion she was given this curative eurythmy exercise which was divided between upper and lower: the said vowels with the legs and the three consonants with the arms, to be performed alternately.

'L-M-O'

For colitis with meteorism (flatulence).

A 43-year-old woman patient who had for many years had stomach and intestinal trouble, together with severe constipation, was attacked by violent and acute colic after several operations. Rudolf Steiner said about the prescribed sequence: 'If this exercise is done successively then the etheric body is pressed together into a whole.'

'L-I', 'M-A', 'R-U'

For liver–intestinal disturbances.

The 48-year-old woman patient complained of unyielding sleep interruption, severe constipation with flatulence, hot flushes, cold feet and very rapid fatigue.

In this sort of sleep interruption, caused by the digestive system, the over-tired patient goes to sleep quickly only to wake again after a short sleep.

In contrast to these conditions there are difficulties in going to sleep which are caused by overstimulation of the nervous system. These patients are unable to free themselves from their conceptions and thoughts. For this predisposition there are other exercises, for example, 'A-Veneration'.

Heart patients also often cannot enjoy uninterrupted sleep. Frequent awakening occurs because of an organic fear arising in the heart if the ego and astral body are too long away from the body. In such cases the 'Love-E' exercise is apt.

'S-M-I-A'

For over and under-functioning of the thyroid gland.

The woman patient was small, pale, puffy, myxoedematous—tiring quickly—and complained of stiffness in the legs and of flatulence. Rudolf Steiner called this condition an under or over-functioning of the thyroid gland, a case of suppressed exophthalmic goitre.

'T-S-R-M-A'

For hayfever (allergies).

The patient suffered besides with neuralgic and muscular pains. He complained also of headaches and periodic occurrences of bladder weakness.

'N-O-R-M'

For stimulating vitality.

The delicate, prematurely aged lady patient had mild digestive troubles.

'L-S-A-M-I'

For obesity (see also Chapter 5).

*

On the subject of curative eurythmy for cancer patients let the following be said: from experience with such patients the inner immobility and rigidity is recognized—their sense perceptions are often very dulled and strikingly lacking in colour.

Different treatment is required for the various manifestations and stages of the illness. Therefore a particularly close co-operation is necessary between doctor and curative eurythmist.

We have only a few specific indications from Rudolf Steiner. Curative eurythmy is certainly of very great importance for those with cancer—

as much in the pre-cancerous stages, as after the development of a tumour, both pre- and post-operative. The person who has a tendency to cancer formation tends to become too much like the earth. 'He develops the earth forces in himself too strongly.' [17 July 1924.] We can counteract this 'getting too much like the earth' with eurythmy and curative eurythmy.

Symptoms are often based on disturbances in the digestive region as, for instance, severe constipation and persistent insomnia. These symptoms point to where treatment should begin.

'L–T–D–R'

This was prescribed for a pre-cancerous case.

We were dealing here with long-standing constipation in a 49-year-old patient who had had various treatments over the years, none of which had been able to effect any lasting cure. His whole digestion was very sensitive—he had severe meteorism. He also caught cold very easily. Through doing curative eurythmy the symptoms disappeared astonishingly quickly. The patient himself was surprised and went on doing the exercises into his old age.

Here was a pre-cancerous disposition, but the exercises can also be used for constipation, if there is a weakness, and particularly when it is in the region of the upper abdomen where the large digestive glands are.

*

If we have to deal with an existing tumour, it is important, first of all, as in all treatment of carcinoma, to convey a process of warmth to the tumour. The generation of warmth comes about through the vowels—the consonants direct the effect to the right place. The localization of the tumour will determine the choice of consonants. The aspect of the formation of the human body as described in Chapter 10 will serve as a guideline.

'O–E–M–L–Ei–B–D'

This was given to a 32-year-old woman patient who had been operated on and afterwards had undergone radiation treatment for cancer of the breast.

From this sequence we can deduce important indications for the treatment of cancerous growths. In the sequence vowels and consonants follow each other alternately. Besides which the vowels, as also the consonants, are paired together in polarity: 'O' with 'E', 'M' with 'L', 'B' with 'D'. 'L–M' we know as a breathing exercise—here they are transposed as 'M–L', which is not without significance. In those who have cancer, inhalation is stronger than exhalation. Therefore we have to activate the breathing-out more particularly, and therefore 'M' comes first.

The patient who was given this sequence was an English lady. With other, German-speaking patients, 'I' was often practised in place of 'Ei'.

People who have had operations for cancer often come for treatment for lymphatic obstructions. These appear especially in the armpits after operation on the breast. Exercises have to be done for these congested, usually cold arms, which warm them and permeate them through and through: 'L', 'M' and 'A' and 'I' done with the hands and fingers are especially suitable. 'Love-E' is a wonderful exercise for this, and, if possible, also *'Ich denke die Rede'*. Our experience has shown that mobility and better scar formation can always be more quickly achieved with curative eurythmy.

Epilogue

In this book we have been speaking about the living word. Sounds—vowels and consonants—are described as healing factors. It is an unusual point of view in our day and age to bring the elements of speech into relationship with physiological processes, and therefore the presentation can only be a beginning, and incomplete.

Vowels and consonants, however, are cosmic forces. Only he who is aware of the fact that the human being is formed and has grown out of these forces will be able to find a connection with this new method of healing.

The physical body is an echo of the World-Consonant. We have seen how the bodily forms are created from the twelvefold zodiac. As the name implies, the entire animal world is evolved out of the forces of the zodiac. In the human being these manifold forces are drawn together and have become faculties.

The etheric body is an echo of the World-Vowel. Out of the forces of the seven planets the movements of the vowels are created. They take hold from within of the animal nature in man and guide it into the human attributes.

In curative eurythmy we turn to these two realms of cosmic forces: the World-Consonant and the World-Vowel.

APPENDIX

Healthy Feet—Healthy Man

Professor W. Thomson makes some extremely interesting remarks on this subject in *Therapiewoche* for December 1960. He is at pains to show in his paper how important it is to have proper footwear, not only for the feet themselves, but for the whole organism. Orthopaedic doctors of the present time are unanimous in agreeing that the root-cause of the collective varicose symptoms is, in many respects, due to bad footwear. During the last 50 years there has been extensive foot research which has led to significant results. Above all, the huge number of people with turned-in toes, flat feet and splayed feet has led to the necessity of studying the many and various biological connections which exist between the foot, and footwear in general, and the whole organism. The author is convinced that through neglect leading to deformity of the feet, the breathing and circulatory organs are affected. 'From the neglect and deformity of our feet a direct biological path leads to coronary thrombosis.'

And so today we get an enormous number of acquired deformities of the foot, as opposed to the ever-decreasing number of deformities from birth. The most dangerous thing about the whole situation is that these foot injuries, etc. hardly cause any pain during childhood and therefore only come to light when there is virtually no prospect of being able to correct them. Even with modern orthopaedic operations it is impossible to achieve complete restoration or recovery. All efforts, therefore, should be directed towards prophylactic measures being taken to prevent these distressing conditions.

Bibliography

Main works by Rudolf Steiner referred to in the text. Lecture dates are in brackets.

Curative Eurythmy (12–18 April 1921, 28 October 1922).
Curative Education (25 June –7 July 1924).
Eurythmy as Visible Speech (24 June–12 July 1924).
Spiritual Science and Medicine (21 March–9 April 1920).
Occult Physiology (20–28 March 1911).
Man in the Light of Occultism, Theosophy and Philosophy (2–12 June 1912).
Wonders of the World, Ordeals of the Soul, Revelations of the Spirit (18–28 August 1911).
The Evolution of Consciousness (19–31 August 1923).
Man as Symphony of the Creative World (19 October–11 November 1923).
Study of Man (21 August–5 September 1919).
True and False Paths in Spiritual Investigation (11–22 August 1924).
Speech and Drama (5–23 September 1924).
Man: Hieroglyph of the Universe (9 April–16 May 1920).
The Easter Festival Considered in Relation to the Mysteries (19–22 April 1924).
Rosicrucianism and Modern Initiation (4–12 January 1924).
The Wisdom of Man (23, 25–27 October 1909; 1, 2, 4 November 1910).
Supersensible Man (13–18 November 1923).
The Effect of Occult Development upon the Self and the Sheaths of Man (20–29 March 1913).
Spiritual Science and the Art of Healing (17, 21, 24 July 1924).
Anthroposophical Approach to Medicine (26–28 October 1922).
Fundamentals of Therapy (in collaboration with Ita Wegman), pub. 1925 (1983 in English).

Works by other authors which have been translated:
Dubach-Donat, Annemarie: *Basic Principles of Eurythmy*.
Baumann, Elisabeth: *Eurythmy Therapy in Practice*.
Wachsmuth, Guenther: *The Etheric Formative Forces in Cosmos, Earth and Man*.

Index

'A', 14, 21–7, 28, 32, 41, 50, 55, 65, 69, 74, 76, 84, 135, 160, 171
  case histories, 27
  for kleptomania, 54–5
  for overstimulation of sexual organs, 24
  for vertical growth, 43
  metamorphoses, 27
'A-E-I', 42
'A-E-I—I-E-A', 18, 42, 59
'A-E-I-O-U', 42, 53, 69, 86
'A-H', 25
'A-O-U', 76
'A-O-U-M', 58, 76
'A-Veneration', 19, 24–5, 48, 108, 161, 168
acids and the astral body, 103, 106, 109
acoustic nerve, 56
acromegaly, 129
acute illness, 20
adenoids, 91, 102
agoraphobia, 167
air-organism, 7, 42, 45, 76, 94
albumenizing forces, 85
alcoholism, 35
alimentary canal, *see* digestive system
allergies, 25, 169
alliteration for left-handedness, 38
alphabet, 11–15
  Hebrew, 11–12
ambidexterity, 39
amoral tendencies, 40
anacidity, 106, 108
anaemia, 34, 64, 107
angina pectoris, 33
anorexia, 153

antimony, forces of, 85
antipathy, 6, 37, 66, 128
antispastic rhythm, 69
anxiety, 29, 35, 62, 99–100, 126, 152, 167
Apollonian forms, 37, 64
Aquarius, 122, 134, 146, 148, 149, 160
Aries, 134, 135, 148, 149
arterial sclerosis, 48
arthrosis, 157
asthma, 45, 59, 84, 85, 92, 95
astigmatism, 38, 49
astral body, 6, 23, 25, 32, 35, 40, 47, 48, 49, 55, 62, 70–1, 94, 95, 96, 99, 102–8, 113, 118–9, 152, 154, 161
  rhythms of, 19, 94
  movement, 14
asymmetry, 24, 38–9, 43, 109, 162
'Au', digestive, 21

'B', 12, 14, 24, 74, 117–21, 140
  for bed-wetting, 132
  for migraine, 20, 24, 120
backwards imagination, for memory strengthening, 54
balance, 7, 35–6, 42, 51
  exercises, 27, 37, 159, 161
ball games, 37
'Ballen' and 'Spreizen', *see* contraction and expansion exercises
bandages, 70, 167, 168
Basedow's disease, *see* goitre
bases and etheric body, 109
bed-wetting, 41, 129–31, 165

bile, 33–4, 109
bladder, 120, 129, 169
blood, 113
  circulation, 6, 7, 8, 33, 34, 50, 68, 74, 75, 90, 91, 94, 99, 110
  corpuscles, 34, 42, 75
  etherization, 110, 113, 133
  pressure, 33, 99
  warmth, 42
  See also anaemia
bones, 8–9, 42, 48, 56, 128
  defects, 157
  formation of, 76, 140
  fractures, 20
bow-legs, 46, 49
bowels, 103, 108, 114–7, 126–7
  disturbed rhythm, 41
  evacuation, 41, 93–5, 114–7
  See also constipation
brain, 34, 38, 40, 74, 111
  damage, 32, 113
  sand, 48
breast cancer, 170
breath
  shortness of, 84, 91, 95
  sounds (sibilant), 13, 100
breathing, 7, 28, 45, 50, 53, 67–9, 84, 93–4, 105, 151
  difficulties/disturbances, 28, 53, 69, 84, 91–2, 95, 99
  exercises for, 45, 51, 53, 56, 59, 69, 95–6, 151
  shallow, 84
  See also inhalation, exhalation
buoyancy, 6, 27, 34, 36, 88

'C', 141. *See also* 'Ts'
calcium, 48
cancer, 170–1
  of breast, 170
  of stomach, 107
  patients, 63, 169
Cancer (zodiac), 134, 138, 148, 149
Capricorn, 134, 144–5, 148, 149
carbon dioxide, 167
carcinoma, *see* cancer

cartilage, 76
chemical ether, 13, 30. 83
chest cavity, *see* thorax
child, 31
  anaemic, 41, 64
  brain-damaged, 10
  Down's syndrome, 128
  dreamy, 57
  egocentric, 65
  full-blooded, 65
  maniacal, 166–7
  phlegmatic, 69
  post-encephalitis, 102
  restless, 117
  retarded, 29, 57, 70, 102, 127, 128, 155
  rockers, 180
  with rickets, 128
  sanguine, restless, 31, 69
  small-headed, 41, 155
  weak-minded, 12, 28, 48, 126
chondrodystrophia (dwarfism), 102, 165
circulation, blood, 6, 7, 8, 34, 50, 68, 74, 75, 90, 91, 94, 99, 110
  poor, 33, 91
  peripheral, 33
climacteric, 67, 153
clumsiness, 29
colics, 101, 168
colitis, 168
colon, 41, 114–7,
  evacuation, 41, 93–5, 114–7. *See also* constipation
concentration exercises, 37, 62
conceptual development, 127
consonant sequences, 151–63
consonants, 5, 6, 12, 16, 17, 69, 84, 86, 88–132, 133–50, 164–71, 172
  and vowels, 81–7
  colouration via vowels, 13
  in imagination, 153
  while standing still, 57
  with copper rod, 162
  with feet, 153,

with head, 154
constipation, 89, 95, 108, 113, 114-7, 126-7, 153, 168, 170
constitution
  fat or thin, 29, 32 44-5
  hysterical, 131-2
constitutional disorders, 18. *See also* obesity; thinness
'Contraction and Expansion', 37, 156, 157, 161
co-ordinated movement exercises, 40-1
copper balls and rods, 51
coronary sclerosis, 33
coronary thrombosis, 33, 51
cruelty, 40
curative eurythmy,
  cosmic aspects of, 6-8, 12, 86, 142
  during pregnancy, 19
  in schools, 19
  tone, 59, 69

'D', 11-14, 37, 41, 69, 108, 113-4, 139
'D'-jump, 113
'D-T-L', 152
'D-T-S', 153
deformities, 40, 51, 86, 133, 164
  feet, 60, 46-7, 49, 53, 173
  gall-bladder, 34
  head, 135
  joints, 54, 154, 157
  kidneys, 25
  spine, 36
depressive conditions, 35, 152
'Dexterity-E', 29, 163
diabetes, 41
diaphragm, 45, 104
  etheric, 30
diarrhoea, 60, 99, 101, 113, 126-7, 139, 140
  morning, 154-5
digestive system, 33, 49, 50, 55, 89, 99, 103, 108-9, 113, 114-5, 118, 121

  spasms of, 32, 101. *See also* gastro-intestinal disorders
Dionysian forms, 64
disc lesions, 35, 37
dizziness, 27, 46, 48, 49, 160
Down's syndrome (mongolism), 128
dreams, 99-100
dropsy (oedema), 49, 91
dumb-bells, 27, 37, 165
duodenum, 33, 114,107
duration of exercises, 18-20
dwarfism, *see* chondrodystrophia

'E', 14-15, 26, 28-34, 43, 54, 65, 69
  case histories, 66
  with eyes, 66
  with spiral, 32
'E-on-the-floor', 33, 45
ear infection, 152
eczema, 92
ego, 7, 18, 26, 28, 31, 32, 33, 34, 35, 37, 38, 42, 70, 71, 98
  and human figure, 134
  and physical laws, 25
ego-line, 36, 48, 62, 64, 161
ego-organization, 7, 42, 50, 152
  and bony system, 50
  and digestion, 108-9
ego-rhythm, 18-19, 70
egoism, 25, 76, 84
'Ei', 21, 60, 170
emotional disturbance, 121
encephalitis epidemica, 161
epilepsy, 20, 25-8, 32, 55, 130, 155, 168
equilibrium, *see* balance
etheric body, 26, 28, 30, 32-4, 70-1, 88-93, 102, 110, 157-8, 166, 168
  rhythms of, 18-19, 70
ethers, 13, 30, 83, 115-6
etherization of blood, 133
'E-U-Ö', 59
eurythmic laughter, 25, 61, 105
excarnation, 40, 53
excretory process, 25

exercises
  basic, 56-7, 61-71
  concentration, 37, 62
  duration of, 18-20
  hygienic, 25, 51, 57, 58, 61-71
  rod, 27, 69-71, 162
  soul, 51, 94
  speech, 54, 59
exhalation, 25, 45, 59, 68-9, 84, 93-4, 105, 121, 151
exhaustion, 20
exophthalmic goitre, *see* goitres
eyes, 28, 38, 49
  astigmatism, 38, 49
  eurythmy for, 2, 38, 71
  short/long sight, 38, 49
  squinting, 29, 38, 66

'F', 41, 129-32, 138, 167
fat, deposition of, 43-4,
fatness, 43-4, 45, 119. *See also* obesity
fats, digestion of, 103, 109
fear, *see* anxiety
feet, 46, 147
  cold, 50, 168
  deformities, 46-7, 49, 173
fever, 20
'Fidget-iambic', 31, 69, 96
fit, epileptic, *see* epilepsy
flatulence, 45, 59, 70, 99, 101, 153, 169, 170
fluid organization, 90, 118
foot positions, 66
forces
  albumenizing, 85
  astral, 6
  centripetal/centrifugal forces, 94
  earthly, 6
  ego, 37, 38
  etheric, 6
  growth, 43-4, 90, 123
  imaginative, 17
  mercurial, 42
  rounding, 82
forms

  alternating, 36
  Apollonian, 36, 64
  circle, 63
  Dionysian, 64
  for thinking, feeling and willing, 64
  for walking backwards, 160
  geometric, 36, 63

'G', 12, 114-7, 143
'G-K-A-I', 53, 165
gait, *see* walking
gall-bladder, 33, 34, 50, 73, 75, 101, 140
gall-stones, 101
gas formation, intestinal, *see* flatulence
gastric ulcer, 107
gastritis, 107
gastro-intestinal disorders, 99, 101, 102, 103, 106, 107-9
Gemini, 134, 137, 148, 149
'General use of vowels', 56-7
glaucoma, 59
goitres, 102, 152, 169
gravity, 6, 26, 34, 37, 49, 88, 95. *See also* weight
greed, 21-4
growth forces, 90, 123
  upwards, downwards, 43-4

'H', 12, 25, 93, 103-8, 137
'H-A', 25, 106, 161
haemorrhoids, 99, 101, 119, 132
'Hallelujah', 19, 63, 108, 161
harmonious eight, 63-4
harmonizing
  of abdomen, 66
  of breathing, 53
  of head, digestion, rhythmic system, 57
hay fever, 69
head, 8, 25, 44, 54, 57, 133, 135, 154, 167
  positions, 66
  shaking with 'M', 125, 126, 154

headaches, 56, 101, 114, 119, 169
hearing, 56
heart, 72-4, 110, 139
   'E' exercises, 33
   disorders, 33, 51, 52, 99, 167, 168, 199
hemiplegia, 10, 17, 40, 164
'Hope-U', 51-2
hot flushes, 54, 168
hygienic exercises, 25, 51, 57, 58, 61-71
hypermotility, 10
hypomotility, 10
hysterical conditions
   constitution (in children), 130, 132
   paralysis, 153

I, *see* ego
'I', 14, 35-42, 59, 84, 156, 160
   for squints, 38
   with stiff shoulders, 37
'I have got hold of myself', 29
'I', 'U', 'E', 60
'I will—I cannot—I must', 62-3
'I-A-O', 19, 57, 161
'I-A-U—with the legs, L-M-R—with the arms', 168
'I-E-Ei', 60
'I-E-O-U-A', 57
'I-L-M', 167
'I-O-A', 58
'I-O-A—L-M-S', 167
'I-O-U', 52
'*Ich denke die Rede*', 65, 171
'*Ich habe mich*', 29
'*Ich will—Ich kann nicht—Ich muss*', 62-3
idiocy, 38
illusions, 48
imagination
   too much/too little, 57
imitation, 18, 59
incarnation process, 23, 46, 53
industrial life, 61
infantile paralysis, 161-3
inflammatory conditions, 44

influenza, 160
inhalation, 25, 45, 68, 69, 84, 93, 105, 121, 151, 155
inhibitions, 152
'*Innere hat gesiegt*', 63
insomnia, 24, 96, 152, 161, 168, 170
intellectuality, 126
intervertebral discs, 36, 37
intestines, 41, 93-5, 103, 108, 114-7, 126-7
   colic, 168
   paralysis, 102, 168
   See also constipation
iron deficiency, *see* anaemia

jaw malformations, 164
joints, deformities of, 54, 154, 157
Jupiter, 73, 74, 77

'K', 13, 114-7, 143
   for stammering, 53
kidney-stones, 101
kidneys, 25, 74, 83, 118, 124
   diseases of, 84, 99, 118-9
   malformation, 25
   radiations from, 25, 119
kinetic disturbances, 24, 112, 166
kleptomania, 29, 54
knees, 61, 144, 156
   pain, 191
knock-knees, 46, 61
kyphosis, 36

'L', 15, 31, 37, 38, 88-93, 144
'L-A', 25
'L-A ', 'L-O', 81, 164
'L-A-M-H', 161
'L-A-O-U-M', 59, 95
'L-I' for spine, 36
'L-I', 'M-A', 'R-U', 168
'L-M', 37, 48, 63, 91, 95, 151, 167, 171
'L-M-N', 15
'L-M-N-R', 152, 157
'L-M-O', 55, 188
'L-M-S', 102, 152

'L–M–S–R', 153
'L–M–S–U', 91, 103, 151
'L–O', 'R–O', 'S–O', 157
'L–R–S–O', 157
'L–R–T–M', 153
'L–R–T–P', 162
'L–S–A–M–I', 169
'L–S–N–R', 154
'L–T–D–R', 170
'L–U–O–K–M', 166
labyrinth, 56
larynx, 105, 136
laughter, eurythmic, 25, 61, 105
left-handedness, 34, 38, 162
Leo, 111, 113, 134, 139, 148, 149
Libra, 134, 141, 148, 149
'Licht strömt auswärts. . .', 65
life ether, 13, 30, 83
light ether, 13, 30, 83
'Light streams upwards. . .', 65–6
lightness, *see* buoyancy
Little's disease, 60
liver, 45, 50–1, 73, 77, 82, 140, 168
'Look around thee', 65
'Love-E', 33, 163, 171
lungs, 42, 74, 75, 82
lymphatic system, 42, 90
  obstructions of, 171

'M', 15, 20, 37, 41, 48, 59, 84, 91, 121–6, 127, 132, 146, 150, 164
  with head-shaking, 125, 126, 154
'M–L–R', 154
'M–N–B–P–A–U', 121, 166
'Major and Minor', 37, 53 69, 160
malformation, 40, 47, 116
  of kidneys, 25
  of occipital lobes, 40
  of stomach, liver, lungs, 76
  of teeth, 116
  rickets, knock-knees, bow legs, 47
  malnutrition, 29
Manager's disease, 33
manic conditions, 35, 121, 153, 166–7
Mars, 33, 73, 74

massage, 95
measure, *see* rhythms
melancholia, 31
metre, *see* rhythms
memory, 102
  picture in brain, 111
  poor, 48, 49, 96
  strengthening, 49, 54
menopause, 67, 153
menstruation, 126
  disorders, 20, 41, 101, 119, 126, 152, 154, 168, 170
Mercury, 74
  staff of, 97, 100
metabolic-limb system, 7–8, 9, 51, 94, 121–2
metabolism, 113, 121–2
metals and the organs, 72, 74
meteorism, *see* flatulence
middle ear inflammation, 152
migraine, 20, 24, 56, 120
mineral substances in body, 47–8, 84, 85
mirror-picture drawing, 40, 41
miscarriage, 20, 154
mongoloid children, *see* Down's syndrome
Moon, 72, 74, 85
morality, 41, 54
motor nerves, 8
movements, 5–10
  guided, conscious, 152, 160
  co-ordinated, 41
  disturbed, 9–10, 160
  involuntary, 5, 49
  restricted, 10
  voluntary, 5–6
muddled thinking, 58
multiple sclerosis, 159–60
muscle formation, 77
muscular atrophy, 58, 59, 158
muscular dystrophy, 158
muscular rheumatism, 156, 169

'N', 15, 126–9, 147
'N–O–R–M', 169

nausea, 27, 153
nerve-sense system, 8, 94, 121, 127
nerves, 8, 31, 113, 128
nervous breakdown, 56-7
nervous system, 8, 12
   overstimulated, 168
   sympathetic, 99
nervous tic, 49, 96
nervousness, 121, 153
neuralgia, 169
neurasthenia, 64
neuroses, 96, 97, 113

'O', 14, 29, 43-46, 153, 156-7
'O-E-M-L-Ei-B-D', 170
'O'-jump, 43, 101
'O-L-O-R-O-M-O', 156
'O-on-the-floor', 45
'Ö', 59
obesity, 29, 42, 43-5, 153
obsessions, 49
obstipation, *see* constipation
occipital lobes, malformation of, 40
oedema, 49, 90
opic nerve, 31
organs, seven main, 72
   formative process and vowels, 72-8
otitis media, 152
otosclerosis, 56
overnourishment, 29, 31, 43

'P', 117-21, 140
'P-T-L-R', 157
palpitations, 99
pancreas, 33, 42
   tuberculosis, 60
paralysis, 10, 17, 20, 60, 86, 133, 150, 162
   agitans, *see* Parkinson's disease
   hysterical, 153
   one-sided spastic, 164
paraplegia, 10
Parkinson's disease, 32, 35, 160-1
pedantry, 31
peewit step, 122, 123

pentagram, 36, 63
peristalsis, 89-90, 101
perspiration, 27, 44
phobias, *see* agoraphobia; anxiety
physical body, rhythm of, 19, 70
pineal gland, 110-11
Pisces, 134, 147, 148, 149
pituitary, 110-11
planets and the organs, 72-4
poetry, 54
   changing rhythms of, 56
poliomyelitis, 161-3
polyarthritic disorders, 112, 155
post-encephalitic disorders, 112
posture, 37, 46-7, 65, 70, 71
pre-cancerous treatment, 170
pregnancy
   eurythmy during, 19-20
   vomiting during, 108
preventive treatment, 18, 33, 94, 107, 170
   for foot deformities, 51
prolapse, 49
prophylaxis, *see* preventive treatment
psychic 'F', 129
psychopathic tendencies, 43
puberty, 123, 124
pulse, 33, 67
pyloric spasms, 106, 107-8
pyloric stenosis, 106
pyramidal tract, 31

'Q', 114-7
'*Qui-qui*', 71

'R', 48, 69-70, 93-7, 105, 136, 166
'R-L-M', 156
'R-L-M-N', 128, 155
'R-L-S-I', 93, 166
'R-R-R-M-B', 158
'R-S-L', 153
'R-S-L-M', 154
reproductive organs, 24, 74, 100, 142
resonance, 16
respiration, *see* breathing
rest, 18

rheumatic illnesses, 119, 155–7
rhythm, 7, 19, 37, 64, 66–71, 94, 96–7, 105
rhythmic system, 57, 93, 121.
   See also breathing
rhythms, 7, 96–7
   alternating, 38, 56
   anapaest, 64, 68, 80
   antispastic, 69
   dactyl, 63, 64, 68
   hexameter, 53, 69
   iambus, 68
   of human being, 19
   of organs, 42, 50–1, 97
   of sleeping, 96–7
   trochee, 68, 69
ribs, 44
rickets, 47–8, 128
right-handedness, 38
rockers, 165
rod exercises, 27, 69–71, 162

'S', 41, 45, 69, 97–103, 142
'S–M', 'H–M', 126
'S–M–A', 'L–M–I', 'T–M–U', 164
'S–M–I–A', 169
'S–R–L–M', 155
'S–R–T', 161
'S–U–L–A', 165
Sagittarius, 134, 143, 148, 149
St Vitus' dance, 24
Saturn, 50–1, 73, 77
'Sch', 103–4, 106
'*Schau in Dich—Schau um Dich*', 64–5
schizophrenia, 57
sclerosis
   arterial, 48
   senile, 48
scoliosis, 36
Scorpio, 134, 142, 148, 149
self-assertion, 35
sense-nerve system, 8, 127
sense perception, 23–4
   dull, 118, 169
sentient body, 70

sentient soul, 70
sexual life, intrusive, 22–3
sexual organs, *see* reproductive organs
shock, 29, 106, 126, 131, 157
shyness, 35
skeleton, 42
sleep, 96–7, 168, 170
   exercises for insomnia, 19, 24, 126, 152, 161, 168
sleeping sickness, 161
'*So-ist-est*', 71
solar plexus, 66, 140
'Soul-O', 43
sounding the vowels, 16
sounds
   breath (sibilant), 13, 100
   dental, 12, 13, 53, 56
   explosive, 13, 108, 114, 117, 121, 126
   labial, 12, 56
   liquid, 13
   palatal, 12
   vibrant, 13
spasm-releasing exercises, 69
spasms, 32, 69
   diaphragmatic, 45
   digestive, 32
spastic paralysis, 32, 164
speech, 11, 136
   centre, 38
   exercises, 54, 59
   poor, 56
spine, 35–7, 44, 45
spiral movement, 71
spleen, 50–2, 71, 73, 75, 140
squinting, 29, 38, 66
stammering, 43, 53, 69, 86, 165
standing, *see* posture
stealing, 29, 54–5
stepping, 35, 61–2, 159–60
stomach, 103–4, 106–8, 114, 119, 153, 168
   acidity of, 104, 107, 108, 109
   cancer, 107
   cramps, 101

pain at puberty, 108
ulcers, 107
Sun, 73
symmetry, plane of, 28, 40
sympathy, 37, 66, 128
'Sympathy and Antipathy', 66

'T', 41, 69, 108-14, 139
'T-I-A-O-I-T', 58
'T-L-R-S', 160
'T-S-R-M-A', 169
taste, sense of, 103
Taurus, 134, 136, 148, 149
teeth, 25, 116
   change of, 124
temper outbursts, 64
tempo, changes of, 18, 37
'The inner has triumphed', 63
'The outer has triumphed', 63
therapeutic drawing, 50
thinking, 39, 56, 58, 62, 127
   chaotic, unco-ordinated, 58, 167
   feeling and willing, 62
thinness, 29-32, 43-4, 45, 153, 119-20
thorax, 105, 138
threefold walking, 36, 61-2
thyroid gland, 169
tic, *see* nervous tic
tiredness, 152
tone eurythmy, 59, 69
tonsils, 91, 102
'Ts', 36, 141
tuberculosis of pancreas, 60
twitch, *see* nervous tic

'U', 14, 42, 43, 46-52, 59, 76, 84-5, 60, 103, 127, 128, 157, 161
'U', 'O', 'I', 60
ulcers, gastric, 107
upright stance, 7, 23, 46-7

'V', 135
varicose veins, 49
Venus, 72-4

vertebrae, *see* spine
Virgo, 121, 134, 141, 148, 149
vitality, stimulation of, 169
vomiting during pregnancy, 108
vowels, 6, 14, 16, 21-52, 156
   and consonants, 81-87
   cosmic aspects of, 72-8
   sequences of, 25, 53-60
   with consonants in mixed sequences, 164-71
   with pentagram, 63

waking, 26, 29, 71, 96-7. *See also* sleep
walking, 7, 35, 50, 62, 160
   diagnosis from, 35, 62
   disturbances of, 64
   on heels, 152
   showing personality, 160
   with stoop, 50
   with vowels, 57
warmth, 77
   body, 28, 77
   ether, 13, 30, 83
   seats of, 45
water
   excretion of, 119
   organism, 42, 88, 119
'Waterfall', 71
weak-mindedness, 39, 166
   in children, 28, 48, 127, 166
weakness in etheric body, 29
will, 9, 44, 68, 136
wind, *see* flatulence
worms, 154,
writer's cramp, 32
writing with toes, 163

X-jump, 46, 49, 89, 113, 115

'Yes and No', 38, 66, 95

'Z', 142
zodiac, 12, 86 142
   and gestures, 133-50

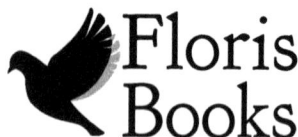

For news on all our **latest books**,
and to receive **exclusive discounts**,
join our mailing list at:

florisbooks.co.uk

Plus subscribers get a FREE book
with every online order!

We will never pass your details to anyone else.

www.ingramcontent.com/pod-product-compliance
Ingram Content Group UK Ltd.
Pitfield, Milton Keynes, MK11 3LW, UK
UKHW021732100225
454894UK00009B/137